WHOLE
BODY
CLEANSING

WHOLE BODY CLEANSING

GAETANO MORELLO, ND

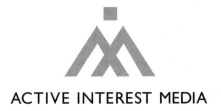

ACTIVE INTEREST MEDIA

Published by:
Active Interest Media, Inc.
300 N. Continental Blvd., Suite 650
El Segundo, CA 90245

Text design by Karen Sperry
Cover design by Silke Design

The information in this book is for educational purposes only and is not recommended as a means of diagnosing or treating an illness. All health matters should be supervised by a qualified healthcare professional. The publisher and the author(s) are not responsible for individuals who choose to self-diagnose and/or self-treat.

Library of Congress Cataloging-in-Publication Data
Morello, Gaetano
Whole Body Cleansing / Gaetano Morello, ND
Includes bibliographical references and index.
1. Health 2. Alternative Medicine 3. Detoxification 4. Toxins 5. Title

ISSN: 978-1-935297-22-2

Printed in the United States of America

ACKNOWLEDGMENTS

NEARLY 2,500 YEARS AGO THE FATHER of modern medicine, Hippocrates, said we should look for disease in the things around us. He believed it was the environment that was ultimately responsible for health and illness. As profound as this belief has become, there something else just as significant—*who we become depends in large part on the people around us.* I have had the good fortunate of being surrounded by some extraordinary people who have influenced my life tremendously. I want to acknowledge them for helping me achieve many of my dreams.

To my beautiful wife, Karlene, who has given me so much and become my partner in life. She is truly the ballast that has allowed my ship to sail to places I never thought possible. To our son Luca Francesco, the little man and the light of our lives. Never did I imagine how life changing having a child could be. It has truly been the greatest experience of my life.

I would like to thank my best friend of 35 years, Federico Fuoco, for his incredible faith in my abilities and his constant support in all that I do. To Dr. Michael Murray, my dear friend and confidant who's brilliant mind has always amazed me. Few people have contributed more to the natural health movement than Michael.

To my brother and sister, Ben and Angela, who have always loved me and been there through thick and thin. I am blessed to have them in my life. And to my father and mother, Francesco and Serafina Morello, who have supplied me with the foundation that is my life. Now that

I am a young parent, I fully understand the sacrifices parents need to make to nurture and raise their children. My parents have been the best of the best. We don't get to choose the family we are born into—I am grateful for being born in this incredible one.

To Kim Erickson my editor for her literary expertise, and Silke Reuthlinger and Karen Sperry for making the book look great inside and out. To Karolyn Gazella—how lucky I have been to have known you for so many years. Karolyn, you really do it all. Thank you for all that you have done for this book and all that you do in bringing the message of integrative medicine to the masses.

And last but not least to Randy Rose, CEO of Schwabe North America. You are truly one of the most brilliant people I have ever known. Thank you for your tremendous support and honest belief in my abilities.

PLEASE NOTE

THE INFORMATION IN THIS BOOK REFLECTS the experience of the author and is not intended to take the place of advice from your own physician. The information is for educational purposes only and is not recommended as a means of diagnosing or treating an illness. All health matters should be supervised by a qualified healthcare professional. You should never attempt to decrease your use of prescription medication without first consulting with your physician. You should also inform your physician of any dietary supplements you are taking. The publisher and the author are not responsible for individuals who choose to self-diagnose, self-treat or use the information in this book without consulting with their own personal healthcare practitioner.

CONTENTS

FOREWORD

HAVE YOU EVER NOTICED THAT MANY people treat their cars better than their bodies? They wouldn't dream of ignoring a warning light on the dash for an oil change or regular maintenance, but they often ignore the telltale signs that their body is in dire need of critical maintenance. What are some of the body's warning signs?

- Do you feel that you are not as healthy and vibrant as other people your age?
- Do you have low energy levels?
- Do you often have difficulty thinking with clarity?
- Do you often feel depressed?
- Do you get more than one or two colds a year?
- Do you struggle with your weight?
- Do you suffer from lack of interest in life or sex?
- Do you have digestive disturbances?
- Do you have dark circles under your eyes?
- Are you constantly hungry?
- Do you have trouble getting to sleep or do you want to sleep all of the time?
- Do you feel anxious or stressed out most of the time?
- Do you suffer from premenstrual syndrome, fibrocystic breast disease or uterine fibroids?
- Do you crave sweets?
- Do you suffer from allergies?
- Do you have bad breath or body odor?

- Do you suffer from chronic post-nasal drip or hay fever-like symptoms?
- Do you have sore or achy muscles?

In *Whole Body Cleansing*, Dr. Gaetano Morello explains that these symptoms may be telling you that your body's ability to rid itself of harmful chemicals – our detoxification system – is being overwhelmed. Furthermore, he teaches us that by reducing the toxic load on the body and giving the body proper nutritional support, in most cases these symptoms can disappear. He also shows us that by addressing these warning signs now we can assure better long-term health and avoid minor problems turning into more serious conditions.

I admire the manner in which Dr. Morello maps out so clearly the problem as well as the solution in his book. That expertise comes from years of clinical practice, helping his patients improve their health. In every respect, Dr. Morello is an excellent doctor. He truly cares about your health and is dedicated to doing all that he can to help you achieve a higher level of wellness. His approach is brilliantly detailed in *Whole Body Cleansing*.

While the concepts of internal cleansing and detoxification have been around for quite some time, their critical role in promoting health has never been more important. We are exposed to an ever-increasing amount of toxic compounds in our air, water, and food. I am amazed that there is literally no focus in conventional medicine on an individual's ability to detoxify substances as a determining factor in their overall health. After reading *Whole Body Cleansing*, you will see what a major oversight that is and you may be amazed as well.

Dr. Morello has seen many patients who knew something wasn't quite right with their bodies, but felt discouraged because they had visited conventional medical doctors who told them that there was "nothing wrong." Often what that means is that these doctors were unable to diagnose a specific disease. Dr. Morello's perspective is different. He knows that many times a body system can be functioning poorly, but be free of recognized disease. In these situations, conventional medicine has little to offer to improve the function of an organ or body system.

Instead, applying the principles detailed in *Whole Body Cleansing* can produce dramatic improvements in your health by supporting one of the most important aspects of good health—proper detoxification and elimination of harmful chemicals from the body.

Our body processes are complex and intricate—a collection of interweaving systems, each dependent on the other. By effectively eliminating harmful toxins from the body, our entire physiology can function much more efficiently. In particular, since a large part of the body's energy expenditure is spent on detoxification processes, lightening the load through whole body cleansing can allow energy levels to soar. Whole body cleansing is a program that can benefit almost everyone—no matter how old you are or what your current state of health is. You can take steps to help your body function better. You can have more energy, feel better, and even look better—all by taking some basic steps to help your body function more efficiently. This simply means following the practices detailed in *Whole Body Cleansing*. It is a tremendous gift you can give to yourself, so enjoy!

Michael T. Murray, ND
co-author of the *Encyclopedia of Natural Medicine*

INTRODUCTION

THE IDEA THAT CHRONIC DISEASES ARE as prevalent today as any other time in history is puzzling. Even with the tens of billions of dollars spent yearly on medical care, are we any better off now than during any other time in our history? The pundits might tell you we are living longer, but others will counter that argument with evidence that paints a very different picture.

Cardiovascular disease—including heart attacks, strokes, congestive heart failure, and hypertension—remains the No. 1 killer. Cancer— including lung, breast, testicular, prostate, liver and cervical cancer—is a close second. As a matter of fact, an article published in 1994 in the *Journal of the American Medical Association* showed that the rate of cancer in men and women born after 1940 was 200 percent and 50 percent higher respectively than in the previous generation.

Diabetes has hit epidemic levels while new childhood diseases like autism and attention deficit disorder (ADD) are quickly becoming widespread. What is going on? Shouldn't we be reducing the rates of these diseases and becoming an overall healthier generation?

The mainstreamers in the healthcare industry will always use the life expectancy argument—that people today are living longer because of the effectiveness of modern medicine. Even during the dozens of interviews I do every year, mainstream thinkers always point to the fact that we are living longer. They'll claim that 100 years ago people only lived to the age of 45, and now the average life expectancy in the United States is about 76 years. They will then credit modern medicine for this supposed increase in lifespan. They use this same justification to explain the uptick in degenerative diseases. It's because we are living longer, they say.

But, people aren't living longer today because of modern medicine. The number is higher because of the way we calculate life expectancy. If we look back to the 1700s, we find a number of famous people who lived over 76 years of age. For example, Benjamin Franklin (84 years), Samuel Johnson (75), Thomas Jefferson (83), and John Adams (91), just to name a few. People lived just as long. The difference was that the survival rate of newborns was considerably lower at the beginning of the century.

To give you an example from my own family, my grandmother gave birth to 10 children between 1929 and 1949. Only five of those children survived. Three of the children, including my father, are still living, while the other two died at the ages of 86 and 67. If we were calculating life expectancy and assumed the rest of the children died in their 70s, life expectancy would be calculated between 42 and 45 years of age. Even though most of the offspring lived to 70+ years of age, because of siblings who died at birth we get a number that's not reflective of actual life span. The life expectancy calculation is skewed by the large number of pregnancies occurring at the turn of the century and the high mortality rates they were experiencing. This does not give us the actual life span because it takes into consideration death at birth which gives you zero years (80 + 0 divided by 2 = 40 years of age). This would then give us the erroneous appearance that people are living longer today than a hundred years ago. The reality is that people's actual life span at the beginning of the 20th century was about the same as it is today.

WHY IS THIS SO IMPORTANT?

This disparity is really at the core of the message I am trying to deliver. We have to realize that, despite the billions of dollars spent on prescription drugs, despite the incredible medical achievements, despite all of our technological advances, we are not any healthier today than we were a century ago. The living longer argument just does not cut it anymore; we need to realize that there are factors at work here that have not been addressed.

What are the facts we can all agree on?

- Something is going on that is affecting human health on this planet.
- Mainstream pharmaceutical medicine doesn't seem to have the answers.
- New childhood diseases like autism and ADD are on the rise.
- Diet and lifestyle changes seem to be correlated with the development of many of today's chronic diseases.
- The rise in environmental pollution may be playing a bigger role than any of us would have predicted.

ENVIRONMENTAL POLLUTION

One area that seems to contribute to a large number of health concerns is environmental pollution. Many scientists are beginning to take a serious look at the effects toxic chemicals have, not only on the planet, but also on human physiology. Could it be that the tremendous amount of chemicals that now bathe our environment are impacting human health much like they have impacted wildlife?

We've known about the possible impact of environmental pollution since the 1960s when Rachel Carson's book, *Silent Spring*, brought a number of controversial issues to the surface. Her plea centered around the tremendous spill of toxic chemicals into the environment and the effects they were having on wildlife. It was her contention that a day would come when the spring would be silent because there wouldn't be any animals left on the planet. At the time she was ridiculed and attacked by the chemical companies and mainstream scientists for making claims they dubbed "outlandish." But, if truth be told, Rachel Carson was an extremely gifted visionary with great foresight.

In the 1990s, scientists studying alligators in Florida lakes that were contaminated with DDT and other pesticides discovered that the male alligators were born with unusually small penises and the female alligators had abnormal ovaries. They also found that the eggs produced by these same alligators did not hatch (something that is still seen today). These serious effects were linked to the pesticide pollution that now is seen worldwide.

How did this happen? Scientists have confirmed that pesticides like DDT act similar to the female hormone estrogen in the body; they have been classified as endocrine disruptors (see Chapter 3). They also found that when DDT breaks down into its metabolite DDE, it blocks the effects of male hormones such as testosterone. As a result, males become more female-like, a scenario that is occurring in humans as well.

For years, the mainstream claimed that DDT, at low doses, did not impact human health. However, a study published in July 2001 by scientists from the Centers for Disease Control and Prevention, as well as the National Institute of Environmental Health Sciences, found that the opposite was true. Published in the respected journal, The Lancet, the research reveals a strong link between DDT exposure and the likelihood of pre-term birth. The greater the mother's exposure, the more likely it is that her infant will be born prematurely. When a child is born prematurely, there is a wide array of possible health problems that may occur later in life. This follows simple logic that what happens in wildlife because of toxic chemicals can also occur in humans.

At the University of California, Berkeley, research scientists found that the most abundantly used herbicide in the world, atrazine, disrupted the development of frogs at extremely low levels of exposure. Again, the scientists found that, much like DDT, atrazine was changing the male frogs, giving them more female characteristics. Another study showed that frogs exposed to pesticides (atrazine, malathion, and esfenvalerate) at very low levels had serious damage to their immune systems, thereby impairing their ability to resist infections caused by parasites. This again is worrisome because we've always thought that low levels of toxic chemicals in the environment can't really cause harm. Yet what we are finding in animal is that these low levels of pesticides are having some rather serious health effects on wildlife.

How much of the human immune system has been compromised because of the same exposures? This is an extremely important question that needs to be fully answered through more scientific research. But, even without the research, we can logically speculate that the effects environmental toxins are having on the immune system are not positive ones.

This is but a glimpse into the world of toxic chemicals, a preface into the frightening fact that this has been going on for decades. There isn't a single, solitary place on this planet where animals haven't been affected. PCBs, or polychlorinated biphenyls, were introduced in the late 1940s as insulating liquids for electrical transformers and capacitors. They were banned nearly 40 years ago, yet they are persistent in the environment and found in places once thought pristine. Polar bears in Canada's arctic carry PCBs in their tissues.

Our planet is now void of unspoiled lands and truly healthy wildlife because mankind has spread waste over every square inch of it. Toxic chemicals are infiltrating the Earth's wildlife and causing much devastation. This same devastation could also be happening to human populations, which may account for the health problems we now experience. It could be one of the most significant reasons why, after spending hundreds of billions of dollars on advancing pharmaceutical medicine, we have just as many health problems now as we've ever had. We have obviously taken the wrong approach. Perhaps taking care of environmental pollution may also take care of us.

GLOBAL WARMING

It doesn't take rocket science to see that we are changing the biochemistry of the environment through the tremendous amount of emissions we are pumping into the air. How people can dismiss this fact is beyond the scope of our discussion. But let's be clear, global warming is not a fantasy. It is happening, and we need to change our ways or it will change our lives.

Thanks to the dedicated environmentalists and politicians like Al Gore who have brought global warming to the forefront, there is finally some focus on environmental toxins. It is through this work that we are able to bring to you this information so that you are educated and aware of the frightening situation we currently find ourselves in. One important initiative is the Toxome Project.

THE TOXOME PROJECT

The Toxome Project was initiated by the Environmental Working Group in 2003 to assess toxic chemical levels found in human beings. There were seven studies in total that tested blood, urine, and fat tissue for hundreds of different chemicals. The results uncovered in these studies were so alarming that it has become a foundation for my presentations.

This project has awakened people to the fact that we are all toxic and that we need to do something about this problem—not tomorrow, but right now. One of the studies tested for nearly 400 chemicals in the umbilical cords of newborn infants. The researchers found nearly 280 chemicals—180 of which are carcinogenic (cancer-causing) and more than 200 are neurotoxic (toxic to the brain). Could this be contributing to the frightening increase in autism, attention deficit disorder (ADD) and other new childhood diseases?

Adults didn't fair any better. Everyone tested, including respected journalist Bill Moyers, had high levels of chemicals in their tissues. This was a wake up call, long overdue. But we can't ignore the evidence any longer; we need to do something about it!

THE INNATE ABILITY OF THE BODY

I have been practicing holistic medicine as a board certified, licensed naturopathic physician for more than 17 years. During that time, I have seen the horrific effects that "progress" can have on human lives. At the same time, I have also witnessed the incredible resilience of the human body. The body is truly the most amazingly intricate, energetically active life form ever assembled. To discuss the human body from the cellular genetic level going outward to its magnificent periphery would be an exercise revealing how much we still need to learn. Yet, there is much we already know about its incredible self-healing abilities.

Yes, the body has a doctor within. It's the healing power of nature—something that has, in many circles, been forgotten, but something that's just itching to get out in all of us. The healing abilities of the human body were known by the earliest of physicians including Hippocrates, the father of medicine. It was the understanding that the human body had an innate ability to heal itself given the right environment. We see this when we accidentally cut a finger, fracture a wrist or simply acquire the common cold. In each one of these cases, our body heals from the injury or condition on its own—as long as it has the proper environment. The apt environment for a cut is that it is cleaned and has a chance to aerate; a fractured wrist needs immobility; the common cold, rest and fluids.

In these simple examples, we see that healing occurs in the body, but only because we give it the milieu it needs. For example, if we kept tearing into the cut daily, that cut would not heal because we keep interfering with what the body is attempting to do. If you don't immobilize a fracture, it will not heal properly, possibly causing irreversible damage.

When we become infected with the flu, it often occurs because our immune system is not on guard or operating at peak capacity. Maybe we have gone through a period of stress, aren't eating properly, and must travel frequently. Taken together, these events can make us susceptible to illness. We are changing our internal environment so the immune system can not function optimally.

Another example is a woman who develops a yeast infection after taking an antibiotic. What happens in this case is that the antibiotics not only destroy the bacteria they were supposed to kill, they also kill the good bacteria in the gastrointestinal tract. These good bacteria are not only important for maintaining a balanced gastrointestinal environment, they also play a pivotal role in maintaining a healthy immune system. The resulting imbalance in the GI tract created the yeast proliferation.

In essence, the internal milieu of the body and the environment the body is exposed to (the foods we eat, water we drink, and air we breathe) is a factor in our overall well being. Of course, this isn't anything new. Hippocrates believed that we should look for disease in the environment, in the foods we eat, in the air we breathe, and in the water we drink.

Twenty five hundred years later, modern medicine is beginning to realize that this foundational Hippocratic concept has merit. Finally we are starting to recognize that the environment—both external and internal—plays a significant role in the overall health of the human body. This may be the impetus needed to move us in a new direction toward optimal heath. This new direction simply involves changing our environment.

DNA IS NOT DESTINY

The concept that our DNA does not dictate our destiny is not new. We've known for decades that if people stop smoking, their risk of lung cancer is reduced. We also know that reducing the consumption of refined sugar lowers the risk of developing Type II diabetes. There are countless other examples demonstrating that changing the environment reduces the likelihood of contracting a number of chronic illnesses.

A great example that appeared in the November 2006 issue of *Discover* magazine dramatically illustrates this idea. The article showed how the environment can influence the human body. The article described two distinctly different individuals—one who was taller and larger than the other. These two people also appeared to have different facial features. Yet, even though it appeared as if these were two totally unrelated people, the shocking fact was that they were actually identical twins! Essentially, identical twins are supposed to be carbon copies of each other, yet these two were far from identical. So, what happened? When the scientists studied this anomaly, they discovered something quite remarkable: These individuals had been separated at birth and grew up in two very different environments. The foods they ate, the water they drank, the air they breathed and the nurturing they received was all different—and it was this difference that changed the behavior of their DNA.

Titled, *DNA Is Not Destiny*, the article reviewed how the environment can impact the body's ability to read DNA. This may eventually prove that the reason some people develop cancer, heart disease, diabetes, eczema, Alzheimer's disease, and a whole host of other diseases isn't because they inherited these conditions, but rather because we live in the same environment our parents did and mimic their behavior.

A 2004 study appearing in the *British Medical Journal* (BMJ) supported this theory. The review article claimed that nearly 75 percent of all cancers are environmentally induced and less than five percent have anything to do with genetics. In cases of breast and ovarian, the percentage can increase slightly to ten percent, but that still means that 90 percent of all breast and ovarian cancers are caused by other factors, not our genes. The BMJ study and numerous others emphasizes the need for all of us to focus on cleaning up our environment, both around us and within us.

THE INNOVATION OF EPIGENETICS

The idea that two people with exactly the same DNA turn out looking different physically and displaying different physiological weaknesses hints at something that may eventually become the cornerstone of how we practice medicine. Epigenetics (how the environment influences genes) could offer new methodologies to help us understand not only what causes many of today's chronic illnesses, but how to treat them.

To understand how these two individuals with exactly the same DNA at birth turned out so differently, we need to first have some understanding of what DNA does. Think of DNA as the words that make up the chapters in the instruction manual on how you are made. Each one of your nearly 100 trillion cells of your body has a copy of this manual. The manual is your genome, which is made up of 23 pairs of chromosomes. Each pair of chromosomes is a chapter in the manual. Within each chapter are sections containing thousands of sub-sections; these sub-sections are your genes. Figure 1 depicts what this looks like.

Visualizing this analogy gives us a glimpse into what may have happened to the identical twins. Just picture for a moment the instruction manual, and let's go to chapter 23, section 265—the section that talks about height. If we read this section it says, "*extend body to a total*

FIGURE 1

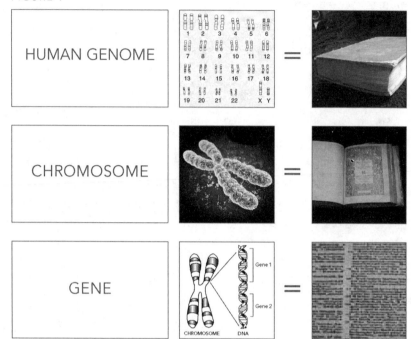

HUMAN GENOME

CHROMOSOME

GENE

height of six feet". Now, for argument sake, let's say that some coffee spilled on the paragraph and now it says, "extend body to *blank*." You can't read it because the coffee stain has hidden the number. Instead, you have to come up with your own interpretation of what the height should be. In the example of the twins, the body of one twin decided to make it five foot ten instead of six feet.

Although this example is simplistic, this is what may happen to your DNA on an ongoing basis. Environmental chemicals are getting inside your cells and marking up the instruction manual on how you should be made. This creates confusion when your body tries to read it. This, in the end, can cause a cascade of problems that may include many of today's chronic diseases.

The underlying message is this: Beware of what you are subjecting your body to because, in the end, it may not only be responsible for the diseases you acquire, but also for the way you look. Taking this a step further really requires an understanding of our own bodies and the environment they occupy. We need to have a grasp of what makes us who we are and what dictates where we are going physiologically. This means having an understanding of our vulnerabilities, our strengths, and our innate ability for self healing. This may sound complicated, but it really isn't; we just need to increase our awareness of what's going on in us and around us.

Our bodies are made up of at least 100 trillion cells, give or take a few hundred billion. The cell is the smallest functional unit and there are many different types of cells making up all of the various tissues in the body. How you feel and how you function is related to how those cells feel and how they function. The quality of your life is predicated on the health and functionality of those very cells. What those cells feed on, what those cells absorb, and what those cells end up retaining is what you become.

WHAT ARE WE BECOMING?

What we are becoming is a receptacle for the nearly 85,000 different chemicals registered with the Environmental Protection Agency (EPA). These are the chemicals found in the food we eat, the water we drink, the things we put on our skin, and the air we breathe. They are ubiquitous (meaning everywhere) and a serious threat to everything we know about cellular physiology.

In the past, physicians and scientists have debated whether or not these chemicals were accumulating in our bodies and having an impact on our health. One example that's been in the news lately is bisphenol A (BPA), a compound used to make plastics. BPA has been found in 95 percent of all people tested. This chemical was first synthesized in 1891 and used extensively in consumer products, before it was shown to mimic estrogen. It is now believed to be a contributing factor to both breast and prostate cancer.

Chemicals are accumulating in our bodies and negatively impacting our health. You would think that things we come in contact with would have been tested before being approved for use. But the reality is that more than half of the 85,000 registered chemicals have never been tested for human safety.

As a result, thousands of the chemicals in our environment are potentially carcinogenic, neurotoxic, and may even be hormone disrupting, (I'll discuss this in more detail in Chapter 4). And we are accumulating these toxins at an alarming rate, creating something called *body burden*. Body burden is the total amount of toxic chemicals in the body at any given time. Estimates have this total at anywhere from 400 to 800 chemicals, depending on where you live and how well your body gets rid of these chemicals.

One type of chemical, polychlorinated biphenyls (PCBs), has been banned for nearly 40 years. PCBs were originally used as insulators for all sorts of industrial application, including the gasoline engine, until they were discovered to cause birth defects. PCBs also cause cancer in animals, suppress the immune system, and exert negative effects on the thyroid. Yet PCBs are still found in our food supply, primarily in farmed fish.

The *Journal of the National Cancer Institute* states that "nearly 95 percent of all cancers are environmentally induced, and only five percent have any genetic link." In other words, the air you breathe, the food you eat, the liquids you drink, and the things that you come in contact with every day dictate 95 times out of 100 whether or not you will eventually develop cancer. This isn't just startling, it's scary! To think that one of the most feared and devastating diseases of our time is triggered by the chemicals around us is really more than just eye opening. Yet, when most people hear this fact, they really aren't surprised. Most people realize that we are living in a time where chemicals are everywhere. In just the last decade we've learned how various toxic gases released in the environment are creating global warming. But the reality is that it's just not the planet that's in peril, so is the human body.

When we look at the fact that nearly 85,000 different chemicals are registered with the EPA and the World Health Organization (WHO) — and that more than 2,000 new chemicals are being added to the mix every year—it's not difficult to see why the health of our world is in peril. As I mentioned previously, the majority of these chemicals have never been tested for their impact on human health. We only know they are harmful because of independent research into their health effects.

You have probably heard about the phthalates found in children's toys and the problems they may pose. Phthalates are used to make hard plastic soft and pliable. They are also used to lengthen the life of fragrances and keep nail polish from chipping. The problem is that phthalates are weak endocrine disruptors and androgen blocking chemicals. This means that, when absorbed into the body, phthalates can either mimic or block estrogen in women or suppress testosterone involved in male sexual development. In a 2005 study, researchers found that, when pregnant women were exposed to high amounts of phthalates, they gave birth to baby boys with a decreased anogenital distance (the distance between the anus and genitals). This supports earlier findings that phthalates can interfere with normal infant male development. A 2006 Finnish study appearing in the *Journal of Steroid Biochemistry and Biology* showed that pregnant mothers exposed to high levels of phthalates had infants who developed a higher incidence of cryptorchidism (the absence of one or more testes from the scrotum). If phthalates are having these effects on infants, what effects are they having on the adult population?

BPA has also been making headlines lately. This plastic stabilizer also mimics estrogen in the body. Scientists now believe that a fetus exposed to excessive estrogen before birth has an increased risk of developing breast cancer during adult life. Recently, BPA was banned from plastic baby bottles. But it may be too little, too late. BPA has been found in 90 percent of the US population tested.

As the old cliché goes, this may only be the tip of the iceberg. Toxic chemicals are on every corner of the planet, and now in every square inch of our bodies. We may not know all the damage they can do but, as a colleague once said to me, "I've seen enough!" Chemical toxins are dangerous to human physiology—science is revealing this fact to us on a weekly basis with studies showing the detrimental effects of things we once thought were safe.

For decades now, many of us have been promoting healthy living through diet and exercise; we have been educating our patients about the benefits of some supplements and the uselessness of others. But, we haven't been as focused on the chemical bombardment that assaults our bodies every day. It is, after all, the greatest threat we face—one that is not only destroying our environment, but also our human physiology.

WHAT CAN I DO?

This is a question I ask about everything in my life. If I want to help an individual lose weight or if I want to reduce their blood pressure, the question is always, *what do I need to do?* It is an important question because it can guide us to the next steps. In this case, the next steps include learning about the toxic chemicals in our environment, how to reduce our exposure to them and ways to enhance our body's ability to get rid of them.

To do this we need to gain knowledge of our body's detoxification systems. I often come across patient who've tried to detoxify based on some system they saw on television or a "snake oil" sales pitch they found on the internet. Gaining knowledge about proper detoxification will help you avoid the scams and focus on the science.

For instance, did you know that cruciferous vegetables (broccoli, Brussels sprouts, cabbage, kale, etc.) not only enhance the removal of toxic chemicals but also reduce your risk of developing cancer? We need to find out which foods can help us detoxify our bodies and incorporate them into our diet. The process is not difficult; it just takes time to understand the body's natural detoxification systems and then follow up with the next steps. And that's what this book is all about. My plan will help empower you to take control of your internal and external environment.

MY THREE PILLARS

There is a phrase that should be ingrained in all human beings across this planet. What people should always remember is that, *the body has an innate ability to heal itself, given the right environment.* If you supply the right environment—in other words, if the body is clear of toxins, has all that it needs nutritionally, and lives in clean surroundings—then the body can heal from almost anything. To get to this level there are three pillars that are very important. They are education, tools, and compliance. Achieving optimal health relies on these three actions.

1. Education

An important part of healing is learning about the problem. We need to understand what causes the problem and what needs to be done to solve it. The individual needs to visualize this in an easy to comprehend fashion so he or she "gets it." In the case of detoxification, this means having an understanding of what the chemical toxins are, where they come from, how they get inside you, and how your body actually processes them. By understanding these facts, you can visualize the steps needed to minimize exposure and improve your own body's ability to get rid of them.

2. Tools

A mechanic can't fix a vehicle if he or she doesn't have the tools. It's the same with a physician. They cannot properly diagnose a pathology without the right tools. Improving detoxification mechanisms require a number of specific tools. They need to be the right tools, utilized correctly, taken in the right dosages, and combined with synergies in mind. This means using the right nutritional products, the right exercise program, the proper diet, and other detoxification procedures to get the intended results.

Far too often, detoxification kits and programs don't have the right ingredients in the right amounts. Some of the constituents aren't in their absorbable forms, so they never make it to the targeted areas where they can make a difference. Some of these products can actually be dangerous because they don't properly bind toxins and don't have the antioxidant levels to deal with the overspill. When purchasing a program, it's critical to make sure it contains the right tools or else you won't get the results you desire.

3. Compliance

Compliance means taking what you've learned and following up with the necessary steps. This is another area where many people fail because they don't do what is needed. However, I have found that when a patient has a strong educational component and a thorough understanding of the toxins in their body, they have a much higher rate of compliance. This is true especially when patients see holistically-oriented physicians who spend a lot of time educating the patient about the problem at hand. The leverage comes from helping the patient understand the issue. This book will help you become so knowledgeable about chemical toxins and their effects on your body that compliance will no longer be an issue.

TO SUMMARIZE

There is little doubt that the toxic chemicals that make up our environment are becoming a serious threat to every human on the planet. If we want to become healthier, we not only need to minimize our exposure to them, we need to improve our own body's ability to remove them. This is something that should be at the forefront of any health program. It is something that we can no longer ignore. And it is the key focus of this book.

1

Detoxification

THE GENERAL CONSENSUS IS THAT THE majority of diseases are linked to eating a Western diet, stress and a sedentary lifestyle. Both mainstream and holistic philosophies accept this fact, as evidenced by the explosive growth in fitness centers, health food stores and weight loss programs—all designed to improve lifestyles and ultimately overall health.

Yet there is another factor not discussed that contributes to our health problems. We seldom see it listed as a major factor in the development of heart disease, diabetes, obesity or cancer. What I am referring to are the thousands of toxic chemical that we pour into the environment on a daily basis. I am talking about the chemicals found in the foods we eat, in the water we drink, in the air we breathe and in the things that come in contact with our skin. These are the chemicals that are now found in every human being on the planet.

The question that has been debated is whether or not these chemicals are having an impact on human physiology. Two of the goals of this book are first, to make clear that we are indeed toxic and second, that these toxicities are having a major impact on our overall health. They are affecting our immune systems, our nervous system including our brains, our endocrine system, and every other biological system. These chemicals are a major threat, yet we know very little about them. Even more disturbing is the fact that we know very little about their negative health effects.

A THOUGHT

How many times have we tried to link fatigue, arthritis or any immune condition to the presence of chemical toxins? If you are like most, the answer to that question will be "seldom." We don't often think of invisible chemicals as part of the health crisis we are now experiencing. Yes, we talk about carcinogens like cigarette smoke as being linked to cancer, but how often have you thought about the bug spray underneath your sink or the fertilizer in your garage? How often have you thought of your deodorant as a possible contributing factor to neurological diseases? It's time to expand our thinking.

In the end we need to understand what they are, where they come from, and how we can reduce our overall exposure. In other words we need to understand how we can get rid of them. Ultimately, the only way to reduce the toxic load in the body is to reduce exposure and improve our body's ability to get rid of chemical toxins.

WHAT ARE TOXINS?

For the purposes of this book, a toxin will be defined as any substance that can have detrimental effects on human physiological functions. Toxins are capable of causing disease on contact or through absorption by body tissues. The toxins then interact with various molecules and disrupt normal biological activities. Toxins can vary in their effects, ranging from minor reactions to those causing instant death. What all this simply means is that toxins are not good for you, so you need to learn as much as possible about them—and how to avoid them.

There are two types of toxins, exogenous (external) and endogenous (internal) toxins. Exogenous toxins are the toxins found in the food we eat, the water we drink, the air we breathe, and the things that come in contact with our skin. Endogenous toxins on the other hand are those produced by various metabolic functions of the body, and by bacteria and other microorganisms in the gastrointestinal tract.

You can already see where most of the toxins are coming from—the environment.

There are literally tens of thousands of chemicals all around us that seep into our bodies. This overloads our body's ability to get rid of these chemicals, thus causing an increase in our body burden.

BODY BURDEN

Although the human body is amazing, it can only handle so much before the burden becomes too much. Body burden refers to the total amount of chemical toxins present in the human body at any given time. You may find others refer to this as *chemical load*. The body burden is determined through monitoring the chemical toxins or their metabolites in the blood, urine, and adipose (fatty) tissue of the people being tested. The number will be influenced by two factors: Your total exposure to toxic chemicals and your body's ability to get rid of these toxins through detoxification pathways. People living in highly polluted environments will generally have a higher body burden. For example, farmers using pesticides and herbicides will have a higher body burden for these types of toxins. On the other hand, people consuming a lot of sushi might have a higher body burden of mercury. It is sometime useful to consider body burden of a specific toxic chemical like mercury, arsenic, or a pesticide like DDT.

Some people will also have optimally functioning detoxification pathways and others may not. These people will still have a body burden, but it will probably be lower than those whose detoxification pathways are not optimal. The difference may be due to genetic alterations, environmental damage, or immune dysfunction.

THE CHEMICALS

Toxic chemicals occur both naturally (i.e., poison ivy or a bee sting) and artificially (i.e., mercury, PCB's, DDT or BPA). These toxins can be inhaled, ingested (food, beverages) or even absorbed through the skin. People are often surprised when we talk about skin as being a route of toxic exposure. Yet the skin is an organ capable of absorption. This is why moisturizing creams disappear as you rub them on your skin. Have you ever wondered where they disappear to?

In medicine, we often use the skin as a way of getting medication into the blood, bypassing the digestive tract. For example, female hormones are often administered either through a patch which adheres to the skin or creams that are rubbed into the skin. Both these routes of administration deliver hormones into the blood.

These kinds of medicines may stay in our bodies for a short period of time before being broken down and excreted by detoxification systems. But continuous exposure to certain chemicals can create a "persistent" body burden. Arsenic, for example, is usually eliminated within 72 hours of exposure while some chemicals like the pesticide DDT can remain in our tissues for 50 years.

It is safe to assume that, out of the 85,000 chemicals around us, we do not know how many of them are part of our total body burden. But, scientists estimate that the human body contains anywhere from 400 to 700 toxic chemicals that have never been studied for safety. This is seen not only in people living in major urban centers, but also those living in rural areas. The reason why they are ubiquitous is because they are difficult to breakdown and thus have plenty of time to get distributed. Distribution occurs through a number of means. For example, toxins can attach themselves to dust particles, travel in air and water currents, and make their way into every known territory on this planet. This has made our planet a polluted place and, in turn, contaminated all living things that inhabit it.

FIGURE 1.1

BODY BURDEN = Total Amount of Toxic Exposure –
Body's Ability to Eliminate Toxins

WHAT IS DETOXIFICATION?

Detoxification, or clinical purification, is a system whereby overall body burden is reduced. As we've discussed, the high level of environmental toxins has created potentially harmful levels in the blood, liver, gastrointestinal tract, and nervous system, as well as the adipose tissue found throughout the body. Through detoxification—which involves minimizing exposure, incorporating various foods and nutrients to support the body's detoxification systems, and utilizing various modalities to loosen bound toxins— one can ultimately reduce body burden.

The body's purification system involves a number of different organs and a complex array of enzymes. They include the lungs, the skin, the kidneys, and the liver. The liver is the body's most important organ of detoxification, having an entire system devoted to this most important process. Not lagging far behind are the kidneys, followed by the lungs and the skin. Even the bones have some detoxification capabilities. They actually pick up heavy metals from the blood stream, minimizing their effects on the circulatory system.

Yet even though we have this intricate system of purification, our bodies are still accumulating toxins. This is occurring because our purification systems just can't keep up with the sheer volume of chemical exposure. For example, if you drink a glass of wine, you may not feel the effects. But if you drink a gallon of wine, chances are you will feel horrible because the body just can't detoxify that amount of alcohol fast enough. The end result is a high level of alcohol in the blood stream causing all the problems associated with alcohol overindulgence.

DETOXIFICATION'S TWO DEFINITIONS

When we talk about detoxification we also have to realize that there a two different viewpoints about its meaning. In the conventional medical world, one would be viewed as toxic if he or she had severe symptoms of food poisoning, kidney failure, allergies or excessive alcohol or drug use. In these cases, detoxification would entail the use of artificial techniques to reduce the levels of toxins in the body—dialysis if the kidneys weren't functioning, chelation therapy for heavy metal toxicity, methadone for heroin addicts, and even pumping the gastrointestinal tract in cases of food poisoning.

Although toxins are toxins, the environmental toxins we've been discussing are more widespread. They affect everyone on the planet and the symptoms are non-specific. What this means is that accumulation is slow and so is the damage. Eventually, these chemicals can accumulate to such high levels that they cause more serious problems. It is much like atherosclerosis (the narrowing of the arteries), also known as the silent killer because few symptoms are felt until a heart attack occurs. Similarly, toxic chemicals accumulate under the radar until a health crisis occurs. Because there are no symptoms until a catastrophic disease occurs, few people involve themselves in serious body purification programs.

The concept of detoxification in the holistic world, however, centers around the idea of improving the body's own detoxification abilities. This is achieved by having a scientific understanding of the biochemical reactions in detoxification and how we can influence their effectiveness. Numerous nutrients can enhance detoxification pathways, protecting cells and tissues from active toxic compounds, and improving the body's ability to eliminate some of these chemicals through the gastrointestinal tract. Other aspects of whole body detoxification involve minimizing exposure and being able to dislodge toxins that have been stored over a long period of time.

In the pages ahead, you will learn about these pathways and what these systems actually do on a daily basis. The hope is that we all embark on improving these critical systems, reducing our exposure to chemicals toxins, and ultimately achieving optimal health because of it.

BACKGROUND

A quarter of a century ago, detoxification wasn't regarded as a necessary step to optimal health by the majority of health care practitioners. I, for one, viewed it as people looking for solutions to their problems in all the wrong places. This opinion was developed merely from observing how unhealthy people on fasts and detoxification programs appeared. There seemed to be something wrong with the practice, something that was causing more harm than good.

My interest in studying cleansing methods was peaked early in my medical school years when one of my roommates, who I'll call Fred, began experimenting with purification programs. When you looked at Fred, you saw a pale jaundiced face with yellow discoloration in his eyes. And, although Fred was only 38 years old, he looked more like 50.

I remember asking Fred how he felt and he would often respond with the same made-up answer, "I feel great." The problem with Fred's answer was that it didn't match his less-than-healthy appearance; he often looked dazed and dehydrated. My conclusion about Fred was simple—whatever he was doing was definitely having an impact on his body. The problem was that it wasn't positive.

One of things you will learn later in this book is why Fred appeared so unhealthy. You will also learn that detoxification can be harmful when improperly carried out. I will dispel the myths of detoxification and give you an understanding of what this process actually entails. Through this understanding, you will be able to make informed choices and take the necessary steps to cleanse your body and become healthier because of it.

SOME HISTORY

Detoxification has been around since the beginning of time. For thousands of years, body detoxification has been a part of our rituals for health and well-being. The Egyptians and the Greeks employed all sorts of interesting methods to remove toxicities from the body. Bloodletting was probably one of the more popular techniques. The theory was to cleanse the body by removing bad blood. This was performed by cutting into a vein near the problematic area. Another method of blood letting was to use freshwater leeches to suck the bad blood out.

One ancient modality that has survived the test of time is the use of enemas. Enemas were not only used as a cleansing procedure, they were employed to treat most illnesses of the time. In the olden days, when someone got sick, enemas were the first option. Although enemas don't really have any scientific basis in detoxification, there is no doubt that they do have some other medical applications. Enemas could be useful in people who are chronically constipated. They can also be used to deliver certain medications to the treatment area.

In the 19th century, proponents of detoxification claimed that the large intestine was a sewage reservoir and that stagnation caused toxins to eventually be absorbed into the body, causing illness. The solutions to this problem were laxatives, purges, and enemas to move stool out of the body, thus eliminating the toxins. This was probably the dawn of understanding on how the body actually dealt with toxins.

Today, a number of systems employ physical treatments like colon hydrotherapy, dietary restrictions including fasting, dietary supplementation, intravenous chelation therapy and every possible detoxification kit you can imagine. Proponents of each one of these concepts have various theories as to why they believe these systems are efficacious. They make claims that your liver will work better, that parasites and yeast will be removed from your gut, and that your entire system will once again function normally. The problem with many of these so-called detoxification programs is that very few of them actually have scientific validation. To have an effect, one needs a number of things to be in place:

- Scientifically validated compounds that have been proven to actually work.
- Correct dosing to match those used in clinical studies.
- An understanding of what it is that you are trying to eliminate.
- An overview of the body's purification systems.

Once these criteria are met, you can have a foundation that may help you expand and support your body's ability to detoxify. Remember, there are only two ways of reducing the level of toxins in your body: Reduce the amount of toxic exposure and improve your body's ability to get rid of chemical toxins.

WHAT THE OTHER SIDE SAYS

On the other side of the fence are the detoxification critics who argue that cleansing is often unnecessary and is based on questionable or disproved scientific claims. The Quackwatch web site describes detoxification as an elaborate hoax used by con artists to cure nonexistent illnesses. To be fair, I can understand how some of these criticisms come to pass. A lot of detoxification programs are confusing, have little science behind them and, in some cases, cause harm. But to paint everyone with the same brush is pushing it a little too far.

The truth is that the body has a natural detoxification system that can be supported nutritionally. We can add things to our diet that help improve detoxification mechanisms throughout the body. This is something that has been known for years throughout the medical community. For example, detoxification enzymes, specifically in the liver, can be slowed and accelerated, thus having an impact on body cleansing. This is the reason why certain prescription medications have warnings against taking them with grapefruit. Grapefruit can actually inhibit Phase I detoxification enzymes, thus inhibiting and/or slowing down the breakdown of certain drugs in the liver. The reason why this warning is given is because the medicine should only remain in the circulation for a calculated period of time. Inhibiting its breakdown will keep the medicine in the blood stream, creating some unwanted effects. So, even in conventional medical thought, there are examples of the role that food may or may not play in detoxification systems.

LOTS OF MISINFORMATION ON DETOXIFICATION

Checking out the latest television infomercial on detoxification really demonstrates the need for education on what this process involves. Exaggerated medical claims and hype make these programs dangerous for the general population. People really need to educate themselves on what detoxification is and how they can actually improve their health with a scientifically-based internal cleansing program.

Something that bothers me is how toxins are portrayed in some infomercials and magazines. Chemical toxins don't look like torturous stored-up feces that resemble fossilized snakes. They instead are microscopic chemicals stored in your liver and the fatty tissues throughout the body. They are invisible and sometimes odorless, and they seep into your cell's DNA, potentially causing disruptions that may have long term repercussions. They are tiny chemicals that may be circulating in your blood stream, causing immune reactions that give rise to allergies. These chemicals can also cause the disruption of your hormones and interfere with the cells ability to communicate with one another.

What we are dealing with is truly a silent, almost invisible killer that can lurk in your body for decades, slowly building up and causing its final damage when you least expect it. Scientists have found chemicals in every human fatty tissue ever analyzed. In other words, we are all toxic and there is no escape.

AN OVERVIEW

Although we will be discussing the process of detoxification in more detail later in this book, an overview may be helpful in clarifying some misunderstandings. Some people can't understand how toxins can accumulate in our bodies. Others don't think that these chemicals are having any negative physiological impact. There are also many people who just don't understand how a product in the marketplace can contain dangerous chemicals. After all, don't consumer products have to go through government approval?

These are all questions people have—I know, I've been asked them over and over again. So let's take some time and go over some of this information before getting into the nitty gritty of detoxification.

First, don't let anybody tell you that, toxic chemicals aren't accumulating in our systems daily. Science has, for decades, known that chemicals in the environment have the potential to disrupt many different physiological processes. Studies have clearly shown that chemicals can negatively impact wildlife and, in turn, humans.

The reason why these chemical are now accumulating at an enhanced rate is because there are more of them. Numerous chemicals are entering the body through various entry points and not being eliminated as efficiently—or as quickly—as we would like. The end result is what we now see—body burdens causing much disruption on overall human health.

Let's go back to our wine example. If we drink a glass of wine with a meal, chances are that we'll feel fine. But if we go and drink a gallon of wine with our meal, we will in fact become intoxicated. If we look closely at these two scenarios we find that:

- In the first case, the body (more specifically the liver) had an easy time breaking down the alcohol.
- In the second case, the body could not break down the alcohol fast enough so much of it ended up in the blood stream. Some of this alcohol went to the brain and impacted the nervous system.

This is the same kind of thing that happens with toxins. Small amounts of chemicals enter the body daily. If the body can't get rid of these toxins fast enough because there are too many in the system, they circulate in our blood stream and slowly become incorporated into fatty tissues. Some of them get incorporated into cell membranes which also contain fat. This build-up may not have notable symptoms in the early stages of a disease like cancer but, as the load increases, it eventually begins to effect biochemical reactions which lead to problems.

THE CELL

A cell is the smallest living unit in human physiology. Nearly 100 trillion cells are found in the human body, making up tissue that create organs that become organs systems that comprise the organism (human being). These cells contain a number of organelles, each responsible for various tasks within the cell.

Since the cell is so complex, let's just focus on cellular energy production and how toxins can impede this vital process. Energy production occurs in little "energy factories" found within the cell called mitochondria. There are large numbers of mitochondria in each cell, with some cells having more than others. For example, heart cells (which need energy every second of every day) have nearly 3,500 mitochondria per cell while muscle cells have about 350. This is a ten-fold difference due to the fact that energy production in the heart is critical for survival.

How the mitochondria produce energy is a complex system known as cellular respiration. Yes, respiration is a word everyone can relate to because it involves breathing. When you breathe, your body takes in oxygen, which is carried to the mitochondria where it mixes with a number of other nutrients and produces the energy molecule called adenosine triphosphate (ATP). ATP is the body's fuel. Without it, nothing could function and we would cease to exist. It is very important that ATP be produced without hindrances.

But toxic chemicals can interfere with the production of ATP. Cyanide, as an extreme example, shuts down ATP production completely, causing instant death. This is why cyanide is considered a poison.

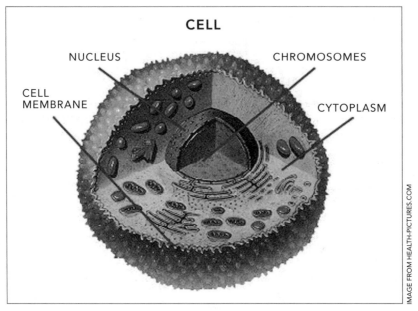

CELL

NUCLEUS   CHROMOSOMES

CELL
MEMBRANE   CYTOPLASM

FIG 1.2 The cell contains a number of different organelles that include mitochondria, the energy producing factories.

Imagine how many other chemicals can have similar but milder effects; perhaps not causing death but leading to a number of other problems. Much of this may be going on inside the body, causing a slow but eventual loss of cell function.

With the advancements in testing and scientific research in environmental medicine there is no denying the fact that toxicities are within every living thing. Science has also begun to discover that these toxicities are contributing to the ever-expanding domain of chronic diseases. Some of the positive things to come out of these observations are the health alerts on BPA and phthalates. Still, we have a long way to go to truly begin saving the planet and its inhabitants.

BACK TO THE BEGINNING...

Why do so many people utilizing detoxification programs look so sickly? This question is one of the reasons I wrote this book—to lay out the science of proper detoxification. In the past, there has been much said about cleansing that had absolutely no scientific basis. I have spent countless hours searching for credible evidence to back up these claims, to no avail. Nothing in the medical literature supports the use of certain herbs to purify the blood or benefit the lymphatic system. The reason I found nothing was because there is nothing to find, just assertions with little scientific support.

This brings us back to the original question as to why some people on detoxification programs look so unhealthy. The simple answer is that they were not undergoing proper scientific detoxification. They were instead moving toxins in the body from one place to another creating something we call oxidative stress. Oxidative stress is like sending out a whole bunch of little bombs to different parts of the body, where they can do serious damage. A more intricate view of this will be explained in the chapter on scientific detoxification.

WE'VE COME A LONG WAY

In the last quarter century, scientists have developed an understanding of how the body actually gets rid of chemical impurities. Through this knowledge, we are now better equipped to make recommendations for choosing the right products for detoxification. This wasn't the case twenty years ago, when some fasting techniques were actually causing more harm than good.

Still today, people working in the detoxification field employ the use of enemas, colonics and other invasive systems that are supposed to clean the gastrointestinal tract with the hope of ridding the body of toxins. In some circles, this is the preferred system of cleansing even though very little research supports such methodologies. But even if science one day proves that colonics are beneficial and free from side effects, this is far from the complete picture of proper purification.

To understand what proper detoxification is we need to look at the science of how the body naturally gets rid of toxic chemicals. For example, how does the body get rid of alcohol, over-the-counter and prescription drugs, and food-borne poisons? We know that these things get inside our bodies and we know that there are efficient systems to eliminate them. If we can understand how these systems work, we can also understand how we can effectively enhance their function.

THE SCIENCE OF DETOXIFICATION

The science of detoxification involves doing a number of things that will, in the end, improve your body's ability to rid itself of toxins and, at the same time, protect your body from the detoxification cycle. You see, detoxification can produce so many damaging compounds that it can cause more harm then good, as was the case with my roommate Fred.

A scientifically-based system involves six different steps to ultimate detoxification:

1. Improve overall digestion.
2. Improve energy production, since detoxification is energy dependent.
3. Increase antioxidant status and glutathione levels in the body.
4. Support Phase II detoxification systems.
5. Improve the ability of the gut to bind bile.
6. Enhance stool movement.

Nothing can happen unless the digestive tract is healthy. All healing happens in the gut, so the first step is to restore gut function and improve overall digestion. Secondly, it is important to produce enough energy because detoxification processes are energy dependent. You also need to improve your antioxidant status since detoxification produces so many free radicals. Free radicals use up your body's glutathione stores, which can lead to health problems. By improving antioxidant status we avoid this problem.

Supporting Phase II detoxification reactions is critical to any detoxification program. This involves supplying the body with nutritional support that enhances the function of these conjugation reactions during this phase of detoxification. This phase is also important because it neutralizes the compounds triggered by Phase I reactions.

Lastly, we need to provide the right amount of soluble fiber to bind the toxin-carrying bile and help propel stool safely out of the body. If we follow these primary steps, we will be experiencing scientific and safe detoxification.

2

Our Toxic World

DURING MY ELEMENTARY SCHOOL YEARS, I was allowed to watch certain television shows after I had finished my homework. One of my favorite shows was the FBI, the long running series starring Efrem Zimbalist Jr. as Inspector Lewis Erskine. One of the odd things I remember was the water bottle dispenser in the FBI offices. During the 70s, bottled water wasn't something I was familiar with since I always drank water from the tap. Living in Vancouver, Canada, back in those days, the water was mountain pure and the thought of ever getting it from a dispenser was the farthest thing from my mind.

But drinking water from the tap is no longer a viable option. Many are now put in a position of purchasing bottled water—some even install home water filter systems. City water is often contaminated with toxic chemicals, forcing people to search for alternative sources.

Most tap water is contaminated, but don't think it's just in the cities. The water in rural communities, especially farming areas where pesticides and fertilizers are widely used, can be worse than city water. My own personal experience tells me that it is much worse, especially if the water is taken from underground sources. No wonder people are turning to bottled water.

In 2008 alone, Americans drank approximately nine billion gallons of bottled water, or just a little bit under 30 gallons for every man, woman, and child in the country. Total expenditures for this luxury were just over $22 billion. Is this a booming business? Absolutely! Yet, it's not clear whether or not bottled water is any better than tap water.

The Environmental Working Group (EWG), a non-profit public health and environmental research advocacy organization, tested 10 best selling brands of bottled water for 170 different contaminants in 2008. They bought the sample bottles from grocery stores and retailers in nine different states. What they found was disturbing: 38 total pollutants with an average of eight contaminants per brand. More than one-third of the contaminants found were not regulated in bottled water. Some brands had levels of certain contaminants that exceeded the legal limits in California, as well as industry sponsored voluntary safety standards.

Some of the contaminants found included disinfectant by-products, caffeine, medications, arsenic, fertilizer residue, and a host of other industrial chemicals. Four of the brands were found to be contaminated with bacteria. To make matters worse, two of the samples contained elevated levels of trihalomethane. Trihalomethanes are a group of chemicals that are formed when chlorine or other disinfectants used to control microbial contaminants (bacteria in water) react with naturally occurring organic and inorganic matter in water. These chemicals have been found to be carcinogenic in animal studies.

After this study, EWG noted that, "Some bottled water is indistinguishable from tap water." They went on to say that the only real difference is the price, where bottled water is approximately 1,900 times more expensive than tap water.

EWG also made some important recommendations:
- That bottle water companies fully disclose all test results for all contaminants. Also, it should be done in a way that the public can easily access.
- Disclose treatment techniques used to purify the water.
- Provide clear and specific disclosure of the name and location of the water source.

So, is bottled water safer than tap water or is it just another expense we can do without? According to this one study, bottled water is not that different than tap water.

But, remember, we are basing this on one analysis of ten brands. There are other brands that do follow some of the recommendations made by EWG. For example, on their web site, Fiji water not only gives a well documented history of their water but also provides independent lab testing and the specific source the water they bottle. This is exactly what all bottled water companies should do so that the public can become informed about what they are drinking.

Tap water is tested yearly and the results are made public. Most people, however, don't access this information. If they did, they would know that, out of 28 samples of tap water tested in major metropolitan centers, 24 were contaminated with pharmaceutical drugs.

In another study, researchers testing deep aquifers used for drinking water found human viruses. This means that our water could become contaminated with any virus including influenza, rhino (cold) virus, mononucleosis and other serious viruses. The implications of this are far reaching and it is something we all need to learn more about.

Water is just one of the carriers supplying an array of chemical toxins. There is an overwhelming array of chemicals coming from places you may not have considered. These sources, and the toxins themselves, are things we need to become familiar with if we are to reduce our exposure and preserve our health.

IT STARTS AS SOON AS YOU WAKE UP

From the moment we wake up in the morning till the moment we go to bed our bodies are constantly exposed to toxic chemicals. Chemical toxins are everywhere—from body soaps to moisturizers, shaving creams to shampoos, and even the toothpastes we use. Even lipstick has been found to contain lead, a toxic compound,

The cereal on your breakfast table may be packed with pesticides while the milk you pour over it is probably laced with hormones and dioxins. Yes, the body is bombarded with toxins every minute of every day. It is an ongoing assault that is causing more problems than any of us ever realized.

When I talk about toxins and their impact on human health, people often think it's a modern day quandary. People are somehow under the impression that, like global warming, it's a recent event. Yet this is a problem that's been around for a long time. The facts have been known since the early 1960's when Rachel Carson wrote her famous book *Silent Spring*, which warned of a time when the vast use of toxic chemicals would negatively impact all life forms, including us.

At the time, conventional science scoffed at her contention, dismissing her in the same way they did those that believed nutritional supplements were essential for good health. Of course, now we know that nutritional supplements are incredibly valuable. Yet during the same period, some scientists were discovering that alligators in Florida were experiencing precisely what Carson was talking about. They were seeing male alligators developing female traits because of the chemical toxins in the water.

As we progress through this book, you will learn that chemicals have an impact on all life forms, including people. When one life is affected on this tiny planet, it affects all other forms in one way or another.

So the question of the 21st century is not whether or not we are toxic, but rather how toxic are we? With what we know today, we can confirm that, from the moment of conception till the moment of our death, every human being on the planet is toxic.

What a sad state of affairs! Irresponsibility has created this burden we are all now confronting. Rachel Carson's warnings, her insights into what was to come were real, yet they were disrespectfully cast aside. They were ignored because big money interests didn't like those ideas, because politicians didn't think it was important.

The way we have dealt with these issues and, in some cases continue to deal with them, is at the root of our health crisis. It is also interesting to note that the drug companies that give us the medication to make us better are some of the very same companies creating many of these toxic chemicals.

THE PACIFIC GARBAGE VORTEX

In the North Pacific Ocean lies a massive area that is a reflection of the destruction humans have created on planet earth. The pacific garbage vortex, is a gyre of garbage located in the Pacific Ocean between 135 to 155 degrees West and 35 to 42 degrees North. Shockingly, it is estimated to be twice the size of Texas. Imagine a collection of garbage consisting of plastic materials and other floating debris of this magnitude now invading our oceans and making its way into the food chain. There is so much garbage in the vortex that scientists estimate that even if we begin cleaning attempts today, it would take generations to get it under control. Do you think our world is toxic?

THE TOXOME PROJECT

To better understand our toxic levels, EWG spearheaded a project in 2003 that became known as the Human Toxome Project (HTP). Much like the Human Genome Project that identified the genes carried by humans, the HTP's aim was to map the pollution in the human body. The goal of the project was to uncover the toxins carried in the body, hopefully giving us valuable information on the potential health risks from exposure.

The project consisted of a number of different studies involving adults, children, and infants. Hundreds of chemical pollutants were tested using cutting edge biomonitoring techniques. Scientists, engineers, and medical doctors tested blood, urine, breast milk, and other human tissues for industrial chemicals that enter the human body, as well as contaminants in food, air, and water. The results were shocking. Some of the pollutants found included chemicals causing birth defects, cancer, and damage to the blood, brain, nervous system, endocrine system, kidneys, and immune system. In other words these chemicals have the potential to negatively affect every system in the body.

In one of the EWG studies, scientists analyzed the umbilical cords of newborn infants, testing for 400 toxic chemicals. While the researchers expected to find some, they were shocked to discover 280 different toxic chemicals in the umbilical cords of these infants; 187 were carcinogenic, 200 were neurotoxic, and 208 were associated with birth defects.

Among the chemicals, they found perfluorochemicals used in nonstick coatings for cookware, dozens of brominated flame retardants, and numerous pesticides, as well as wastes from burning coal and gasoline.

To think that newborns are exposed to this kind of body burden is alarming. How could we have predicted such an outcome and, more importantly, what steps need to be taken to change it? Education is a key element. Bringing this information to the public so expectant mothers or those wanting have children can take steps to reduce overall body burden.

Another concern—what are the long term affects on these children? The reality is that we really don't know. However, logic tells us that, since these chemicals have been linked to cancer, neurological dysfunction, and birth defects, we should be concerned. Is the evidence strong enough to link this chemical exposure to autism and ADD? From a purely scientific perspective, probably not, but from a speculative progressive approach, I would think so.

In another study appearing in the *American Journal of Public Health*, 70 percent of four-year-olds in Michigan carried DDT in their bodies while over 50 percent harbored PCBs. DDT is a pesticide which was banned in the United States in 1972 because of its cancer-causing properties. Yet, DDT is regularly found in the fatty tissue of animals, birds, fish, and children. In this particular study, the researchers found that breast-feeding was a primary source of exposure.

Then there is BPA. An analysis of American women found that 95 percent of those studied had accumulated BPA in their bodies. BPA has now been linked to breast cancer in women and prostate cancer in men.

Researchers conducting the EPAs National Human Tissue Survey (NAHTS) have been analyzing adipose tissue from autopsies and patients going through elective surgeries since 1976. In the individuals tested over the last 30 years, the researchers have found styrene, 1,4 dichlorobenzene, PCB's, xylene, ethylphenol, and dioxins in 100 percent of the cases, while 50 other chemicals were found in the majority of the subjects studied.

We've just skimmed the surface of a long list of facts confirming that toxic chemicals are finding their way into our bodies. The theory by some that we are more than capable of handling these toxins is just not true. Toxins are permanently residing in our physiology because the ability of the body to remove them seems to be overwhelmed by the sheer volume of the intake.

The truth is that these toxins are causing untold health problems; it's ridiculous to think differently. We need to realize this fact and begin the process of change, both around us and within us. There is no time to waste, we must move quickly and we must move now.

HOW DID THIS HAPPEN?

What has happened in the last half century to cause this predicament? The answer to this question is at the heart of the problem. It is part of a cascade of events that has transformed our pristine world into a toxic dump that now contains our environmental mistakes.

To start, let's look at a common family of well-known toxins that are found throughout the planet. PCBs were introduced in the late 1940s as insulating liquids for electrical transformers and capacitors to improve safety. Their use spread to plasticizers in building sealants and added to outdoor paint to improve stability. As time went on PCBs became very widespread. However by the early 1970s, scientists began finding them in places from where they had never been used. They were found as far up as the Canadian arctic and all around the Great Lakes. What scientists eventually discovered was that PCB's were not only environmentally persistent chemicals, they actually interfered with important body hormonal functions.

Environmentally persistent chemicals refer to the fact that chemicals like PCB's are not biodegradable like the banana peel you can throw in your compost pile. Their chemical structure remains intact and can therefore persist and be carried by weather, water, and animals from one place to the next. This becomes a problem when persistent chemicals cover our entire planet and enter the food chain. For example, the Great Lakes have been heavily contaminated with PCBs from industrial sources, leaking electrical equipment, and landfills. Researchers have observed that salmon in the Great Lakes have goiters (enlargement of the thyroid gland) and have trouble reproducing.

Studies of children born to mothers who ate fish from the Great Lakes at least two times per month found that the PCB levels in these mothers was higher than in women who did not eat these fish. Their infants were born with abnormally small heads and showed signs of abnormal neurological development. When they were 11 years old, the exposed children had significantly lower IQ scores and were twice as likely to be two years behind their peers in their level of reading comprehension.

How many people consume salmon and other fish, not only from the Great Lakes but from other sources that have been contaminated with PCBs? Research shows that a large percentage of the population tested carry PCBs. In other words, these toxic chemicals are not only persistent in the environment, but also in our bodies.

One of the most frustrating things about these toxins is that they are allowed to be manufactured without extensive studies. As a result, our future pays an enormous price for these mistakes. Who should be responsible for this incredible injustice to our world?

Many say that it is the chemical companies who don't reveal everything they know about these toxins, while others blame government for not protecting us. In truth there is plenty of blame to go around, from the scientists who create the chemicals, to the government officials who turn a blind eye and even to consumers who demand them.

Of course, PCBs aren't the only toxic chemicals found in our environment. There are literally thousands more. Most of the fish we buy contain toxic levels of mercury because we use our oceans as dumping grounds. The home you live in has hundreds and hundreds of chemicals that most likely make up the air you breathe daily.

It is plausible to assume that, because these chemicals are present in such numbers, human physiology has been so compromised that it's not only affecting the function of individual cells in the body, but also our very genes.

As you begin learning more about environmental medicine, global warming, and detoxification, you will become extremely upset and frustrated. You'll be upset about how lenient government agencies have been in allowing so many industrial pollutants to be used without testing. You'll be upset by the fact that most of these chemicals haven't been analyzed for their safety on human physiology. You'll be upset that they haven't been tested for interactions when mixed together.

You'll be frustrated because many of the chemicals in the environment are persistent and just won't go away. They will remain for generations, causing continued damage to all life forms. This is all because caution was never taken; because human interests are always second to business interests.

We've allowed too many untested chemicals to be poured into the environment without proper assessment. Remember, less than half of the 85,000 chemicals registered with the EPA have ever been tested for human safety. If stricter guidelines would have been implemented—guidelines that ensure the safety of chemicals—many of these chemicals would not have made it to market. This would have protected us and, in turn, protected our environment. It seems so simple, so logical. How did they miss it?

BISPHENOL A: A PERFECT EXAMPLE

Another good example of this folly is BPA, which we have talked about earlier. BPA was discovered in 1891 and for decades considered safe. Yet, after all these years of use, BPA has recently been linked to breast cancer, prostate cancer, neurological harm, and developmental problems in infants. The threat is so real that both Canada and Europe have banned BPA from being used in baby bottles.

How BPA's dangerous side was revealed is another interesting story. University of Missouri-Columbia scientists, Frederick Vom Saal and Wade Welhons, first pointed out that BPA acted as an artificial estrogen, causing changes in the prostates of mice. Not surprisingly, both these scientists were heavily ridiculed by the chemical companies. It became so serious that, according to Vom Saal, when Dow Chemical Company—a major manufacturer of BPA—showed up at his Missouri lab, he was told to stop making public declarations about the dangers of BPA—or else.

Fortunately, their threats backfired, and Vom Saal and Welhons pushed even more aggressively with their research. The end result was the discovery that miniscule amounts of BPA act as estrogens in the body, leading to the development of breast cancer in female mice and prostate cancer in males.

At the end of 2006, the National Toxicology Program—an inter-agency body that assesses human's toxins for the federal government—took the position that low doses of BPA may effect "development of the prostate gland and brain, and cause behavioral effects in fetuses, infants, and children."

This damage should have been known before BPA was used to make industrial and consumer products. It wasn't because not enough pre-market research had been done on its safety. When scientists did uncover the possible dangers, the chemical companies tried to suppress the information. So this then begs the question: How many other registered chemicals are also potentially harmful to the body?

WHERE WE ARE NOW

The world has become a dumping ground for tens of thousands of toxic chemicals found in everything from cosmetics to detergents to pesticides to fuels to the food we consume. Factories, power plants, automobiles, and other sources spew all sorts of chemical toxins into the air creating hundreds of millions of tons of pollution yearly. In the

U.S. alone, according to the EPA's Toxic Release Inventory, we have well over four billion pounds of toxic chemicals released into the environment annually. We should point out, however, that the companies volunteering this information do not include the cheaters who are illegally dumping not only registered chemicals but also restricted ones.

As we have learned, our entire world is toxic, from the South Pole all the way to its counter part in the north. What is interesting and disturbing about this fact is that many think it's only our planet that's affected and that somehow humans are immune to toxic chemicals. Nothing can be further from the truth; all living creature are connected and affected.

We need to realize this fact, because only through realization can actions be taken to slow this process and hopefully save our planet and in turn the life forms that inhabit it.

3

Toxin Infiltration

AS I'VE MENTIONED, THE NUMBER OF toxins circulating throughout our planet is vast. Obviously we can't cover every single one of them in this one book, but identifying some of the major players can be useful. A key component of detoxification is minimizing exposure; and we can't reduce exposure if we don't know the chemical or its source. In this chapter, you will gain a better understanding of what these chemicals are and how they affect your health. You'll become better equipped at minimizing your exposure to them.

THE MAJOR CARRIERS OF TOXIC CHEMICALS

When we think of the chemicals that are in the body, it's important to understand exactly how they get there. This is one of the first steps in learning how to reduce exposure. For example, if you know what poison ivy looks like, and you know where it is in the forest, then you'll know how to avoid it. The same thing can be said for toxic chemicals. If you know what they are, and more importantly where they are located, you'll have a better chance of avoiding them.

Toxic chemicals make their way into our bodies through four major carrier systems:

- The air we breathe.
- The water we drink.

- The food we eat.
- The products that come in contact with our skin (creams, soaps, etc.).

Let's take a closer look at each of these.

THE AIR WE BREATHE

The air we breathe is polluted with toxic chemicals coming from factories, power plants, automobiles and a number of other sources. Toxic air pollutants are defined as substances in the air that can cause harm to humans and the environment. These pollutants can be in the form of solid particles (dust, etc.), liquid droplets (rain, snow), and gases.

The majority of air pollutants are classified as primary. This basically refers to substances directly released into the air. Secondary pollutants are not as prominent. This refers to pollutants that are not emitted directly but instead formed in the air when primary pollutants react with each other or with other things floating in the air.

Primary pollutants include carbon monoxide (from vehicle emissions), sulfur dioxide (industrial processes), nitrogen dioxide (high temperature combustion processes), volatile organic compounds (VOC's, including methane and non-methane gas, toluene, benzene, and xylene), toxic metals (lead, cadmium, and mercury), perchloroethylene (from dry cleaning facilities), chlorofluorocarbons, and ammonia. All of these toxic chemicals are emitted into the air every day. Some major sources of this outlay come from the thousands of factories that spew more than 25 tons of these toxic compounds every year. These factories include chemical plants, steel mills, oil refineries, and hazardous waste incinerators. When you combine the total amount from all of these industries, you get millions of tons of waste entering our air and causing an unbelievable amount of damage.

IN NEED OF SOME FRESH AIR

When we think about pollution we always seem to think that it's outside. But the truth is that there are far more toxic chemicals indoors than there are in the great outdoors. It has been estimated that the average home contains about 100 pounds of hazardous material. That's anywhere from three to 10 gallons of chemical waste. This may include paints, paint thinners, air fresheners, carpet deodorizers, mothballs, oven cleaners, drain openers, pesticides, and a whole array of other products. In the past our mindset has been that these products were hazardous to the environment. In reality, they are even more hazardous to our vulnerable human physiology.

The carpeting inside our homes is a good example of this indoor pollution. It emits over 200 volatile chemicals that we are continuously breathing in. Some of these chemicals include formaldehyde, toluene, benzene, acetyldehyde, xylene, phenol, benzaldehyde, chlorobenzenes, styrene, and many more. Styrene alone has been shown to produce neurotoxicity and respiratory illness while formaldehyde is classified as a probable human carcinogen. The rest of the chemicals in carpeting aren't going to do you any favors either.

Maintaining that carpeting can also be toxic. A study of carpet workers showed an increased risk of cancers, including leukemia, because of their exposure to these chemicals. When carpet cleaners shampoo your carpets, they'll often advise you against sleeping in the room that was cleaned because of the high levels of chemicals being released.

One of the major problems with viewing toxins as dangerous is that we traditionally pictured ourselves as impermeable to them. We believed that the only way they could cause harm is if we ingested them. But we now know that toxins can be absorbed by the skin or through inhalation. When you walk down the detergent aisle at your neighborhood grocery store, those "spring fresh" fragrances are being taken into your body. When you apply a moisturizer to your skin, it is absorbed and will eventually make its way into your blood stream.

INDOOR DISEASE

There are so many toxic substances inside our homes and offices that there is even a disease named for it—sick building syndrome. Sick building syndrome refers to a number of symptoms that have been linked to a person's home or workplace including eye irritation, headaches, nausea, and fatigue, as well as odor and taste sensations. The consensus is that these are caused by polluted air inside the building due to a number of contributing factors. Individuals with a weakened immune system or sluggish detoxification can be especially prone to sick building syndrome. Unfortunately, it has become more common than ever before.

Heating and air conditioning units may be emitting a variety of chemicals including mold that could be causing these symptoms. Another probable cause are the toxic chemicals used inside the building or home including volatile organic solvents, sealers, and glues used by builders, as well as the chemicals used to make carpeting and furniture.

THE WATER WE DRINK

The most important nutrient on this tiny planet is water. You can go without food for weeks, but you can't go without water for more than three days. The human body is anywhere from 55 to 78 percent water depending on body size. To function properly, it requires three to five liters of water per day, depending on activity level and outside temperature.

When we look at sources of water, we find that the majority of them are not fit to drink. We find that lakes and rivers are contaminated with agricultural run-off and sewage. Well water contains toxins from landfills. Recent research shows that viruses are also making their way into ground water.

What we have is a situation where our disregard for nature has contaminated our most precious natural resource. Very few places in the world have clean water. Most of it has to be purified and treated before it can be consumed. And therein lies another problem— some of the chemicals used to treat municipal water have been shown to cause more harm than good. Fluoride is a prime example.

THE FLUORIDE PROBLEM

Fluoride is a chemical added to drinking water and toothpaste to help prevent tooth decay. According to its proponents, fluoride is completely safe. But calling fluoride safe is not exactly accurate.

According to the National Research Council, drinking fluoridated water may cause dementia in adults and low IQ in children. This claim was backed by recent studies involving research teams from Brazil, China, India, Italy, Mexico, and the United States. The researchers conducted three studies investigating the impact of fluoride on children's IQ and several other studies on fluorides effects on learning, memory, and behavior. The studies were conclusive that fluoride, at levels of 5-9 ppm, have a negative impact on performance, verbal skills, and full IQ scores. What's scary is that some municipal water levels are within these ranges.

A review presented by Harvard scientists Philippe Grandjean and Ana Choi stated, "In humans, only five substances have so far been documented as developmental neurotoxicants: Lead, methylmercury, polychlorinated biphenyls, arsenic, and toluene. From this evidence, including our own studies on some of theses substances, parallels may be drawn that suggest that fluoride could well belong to the same class of toxicants, but uncertainties remain."

Between 1986 and 1997, a national survey of over 39,000 U.S. school children found no significant differences in tooth decay between children drinking fluoridated versus non-fluoridated water. In fact, evidence suggests that fluoridation can be harmful. Many scientists, doctors, and public health professional are calling for a halt on water fluoridation programs across the United States. In 2005, over 7,000 of them asked the EPA to recognize fluoride as a serious carcinogen in people. Yet, fluoride is still being added to municipal water supplies.

THE FOOD WE EAT

Food provides important macro and micro nutrients essential for life. In their natural and unspoiled states they are healthy for our bodies. However, when they are processed and contaminated with pesticides and herbicides, they carry toxicities that can be damaging to human physiology.

When we talk about food contaminants, we are referring to a number of different pollutants that make up the foods we eat. There are pesticides, herbicides, fertilizers, and many other chemicals found in the fruits, vegetables, and grains we consume. Fish can contain high levels of mercury while shellfish may have a number of organisms that can produce intestinal toxins. Many processed foods contain numerous preservatives, flavoring agents, and coloring chemicals that have been found to be toxic.

Meats are usually tainted with hormones and growth factors that are also finding their way into our bodies.

Many people develop allergies to various foods because of the damage some of these foods create in the digestive tract. An example I often give is gluten sensitivity. Gluten is a protein found in grains like wheat and barley that acts like glue holding the grain together. When people have serious gluten sensitivity, they can develop celiac disease. This condition changes the structure of the intestinal mucosal lining, creating enormous problems in digesting and absorbing nutrients. Foods harboring toxic chemicals may also act on the gut lining causing damage and inflammation.

Over a life time the average American consumes more than 50 tons of food. For meat eaters this could include about 2,450 chickens, 118 turkeys, 33 pigs, and 12 cows. For many of us, this total could also include about 6,500 hot dogs, 20,000 M&M's, 35,000 cookies, 70,000 cups of coffee and 1,800 McDonald meals. That's just a rough estimate! How much of this food contains pesticides, artificial flavors, coloring agents, unhealthy fats, sugar, toxic metals, and other ingredients that have negative consequences to human physiology?

If we analyze the meat alone, we'll find artificial hormones used to fatten up the animals and speed maturation. Chickens and cattle are injected with these artificial compounds to get them to market as quickly as possible. The problem with this is that these hormones are carried in the meat that will be eaten by consumers. Once in the human body, these hormones become incorporated into fatty tissue and may become active. As these hormones accumulate, they may disrupt the body's natural hormone systems. There is even preliminary evidence that these environmental hormones may be a contributing factor to the obesity epidemic.

There are estimates that claim that 80 percent of U.S. foods contain pesticides. That means that most of the foods you are eating contain trace amounts of chemicals used to destroy pests. Pesticides kill by effecting the nervous system and genetic material. Do you think they could do the same thing in your body?

While listening to a recent national news report, I heard the broadcaster commenting on how new evidence suggests there is no nutritional difference between organic foods and regular pesticide treated foods. Who cares! The idea of eating organic is not with nutritional value folks, it has to do with minimizing exposure by reducing the amount of pesticides and other toxic chemicals found in foods. I highly recommend the organic lifestyle, because these foods contain much lower levels of these dangerous chemicals. And don't think it's a hoax; organic foods are now regulated and you can have a level of assurance that you are purchasing better produce that is certainly healthier for you.

THE THINGS WE TOUCH

When we think of our skin, we don't typically think of it as an organ. We often view the skin as covering, creating a barrier that protects our tissues from the external world. But the reality is that the skin is indeed an organ. In fact, it's the largest organ of the human body.

Now just think about all the things that come in contact with your skin. The water you wash your face and shower with everyday and the water in your neighborhood swimming pool. Do these sources of water contain toxins? Probably. These chemicals accumulate over a period of time and can negatively affect the nervous system, disrupt your hormones, and may even cause cancer. Even the backyard playground that your children touch can be toxic.

To get an idea of how things are transmitted into the skin from unlikely places let's look at pressure-treated wood and children. In 2001, EWG published a report called, "Poisoned Playground." In this report they analyzed the arsenic content of pressure-treated wood found in playground equipment, picnic tables, decks, fences, and basically any outdoor use of lumber.

Now you have to understand that most lumber sold for outdoor uses in the United States is pressure-treated. This means that the wood is injected with a vast array of toxic chemicals to help protect it from termites. The most commonly used wood preservative in the United States is chromated copper arsenate (CCA). CCA is a chemical preservative containing chromium, copper, and arsenic. It protects wood from rotting due to insects and microbial agents.

CCA has been used to treat wood since the 1940's. It became a popular way to treat outdoor wood, including children's playground equipment, in the 1970s. Remember that arsenic is classified as a known human carcinogen by both the EPA and the World Health Organization—and children are at greater risk from arsenic exposure because they can't detoxify it as quickly.

According to the EWG report, "an average five-year-old child playing less than two weeks on a CCA-treated play set would exceed the lifetime cancer risk considered acceptable under federal pesticide law." In other words, kids that play on these types of playground are accumulating more arsenic in their blood stream in a short period of time than we would in a lifetime.

The good news is that, after much pressure from government agencies, CCA was finally banned December 31, 2003. The law states that no wood manufacturer may treat wood with CCA for residential uses, including children's playground sets, with certain exceptions. The bad news is that older playground sets and homes before 2003 may still have CCA-treated wood. The next time you are near treated wood, be aware that it may have been treated with CCA.

PERSONAL CARE PRODUCTS

How many times have you applied a moisturizer, sun tan lotion, lipstick, after shave lotion, deodorant or other personal care product to your body and face? If you're like most, you probably use personal care products daily—sometimes even multiple times in a day. Have you ever wondered what happens when you apply a moisturizer to your skin? As you rub the cream into your skin, it gets absorbed and eventually ends up in your blood stream. The problem is, the majority of these products contain ingredients that may not be beneficial for your health.

In a six month investigation into the health and safety of more than 10,000 personal care products, EWG found some major gaps in the regulatory safety for these products. The evaluation compared the ingredients in 7,500 products against government, industry, and academic lists of known suspected chemical toxins. You can visit the EWG web site (www.ewg.org) and review its online rating system that ranks products for their potential health risks and the absence of basic safety evaluations. To get you started, here are a couple of examples to give you an idea of the some of the hazards of personal care products:

PHTHALATES: Concerns about the health impact of phthalates continue to grow as an increasing number of studies link high levels of these compounds with feminization in baby boys. Recent government-funded research at the University of Rochester associated prenatal phthalate exposure with shortened anogenital distance (AGD). Researchers found that the higher the exposure the mother had to phthalates, the more likely the scientists were to find a shortened AGD. When this happened, the boys were more likely to have incomplete testicular descent and smaller penises. What does this have to do with personal care products? Independent laboratory analysis have found phthalates present in 70 percent of personal care products including deodorants, shampoos, moisturizers, hair mousse, and fragrances.

When chemical companies are approached with this data, they claim that the levels of phthalates are so low they could not have an impact on human physiology. But we are not talking about single exposure; we are talking about long term use and bioaccumulation. What kind of body burden levels do we acquire from long term exposure to phthalates?

Common sense tells us that, if we are continuously being exposed to phthalates and thousands of other chemical on a daily basis, the body's ability to get rid of them is compromised. This creates the possibility that phthalates levels in the body are accumulating, eventually reaching levels that could cause harm.

LEAD: When you think of the places where toxins would be lurking, lipstick probably isn't one of them. Yet in a recent report entitled "A

Poison Kiss: The Problem of Lead in Lipstick," researches again found problems with personal care products. An independent laboratory testing initiated in 2007 by the Campaign for Safe Cosmetics found that two-thirds of the 33 lipstick samples tested contained detectable levels of lead. Half of those were above the legal lead limit in candy. (Lead is a potent toxin to the nervous system and is linked to a number of reproductive problems. Children are especially vulnerable to it. The government has put limits lead in candy because of its ingestion by children.) Some of this lead found in lipstick will make its way into the blood stream and possibly start accumulating in tissue.

KEY TOXIC CHEMICALS

According to the EPA, of the thousands of synthetic chemicals registered worldwide less then half have ever been tested for potential toxicity in humans. For the most part, we don't know what these chemicals are doing to the human body. It's absolutely mind-boggling that there are no scientific studies validating that these chemicals are safe. Nevertheless, most people are under the assumption that the household cleaning agents, toothpastes, deodorants, and fertilizers we use are safe because they are available for purchase. We think that somebody is looking out for our best interests before these products come to market.

We put trust in our government agencies. We assume because it's on the shelf for sale, that it has passed safety testing and we can use it without risk. Of course, these are the same government agencies that allow cigarettes be sold to millions of people, even though we know they cause cancer. The truth is that our world has become what we have become, a dumping ground for products that are dangerous for our health and ultimately dangerous for the environment we inhabit.

POUNDS AND POUNDS OF PESTICIDES!

For some perspective, there are over four billion pounds of pesticides used annually in the United States. That equates to just over 10 pounds of pesticides for every man, woman and child. The EPA estimated that nearly 90 percent of all U.S. foods contain pesticides. These pesticides have been linked to hormone imbalances, cancer, neurological diseases, and autoimmune diseases.

There was a time in my life when I thought that farming communities were the healthiest of places. After all, aren't farms isolated from the big cities, free of polluting industrial buildings, and just full of wide open spaces? The reality, however, is actually very different from what I imagined.

My wife comes from a great farming community. Her family has nearly 10,000 acres of land where they grow barley, lentils, wheat and durum. They use thousands of pounds of pesticides, herbicides, and fertilizers yearly, as do all the farmers, in order to have good crop yields. But the consequences of such practices are sad, to say the least. My wife's father died of bladder cancer at the age of 42. Her mother has fibromyalgia. Her sister has thyroiditis and her brother, who is only 27, has rheumatoid arthritis. My wife has been able to control her own autoimmune condition since she moved away from the farm nearly 13 years ago.

This is a personal and unscientific peek into the world of chemicals and their effects on the body. We have no evidence proving that, in my family's case, this was the cause of their conditions. But I can assure you that this is exactly what science suggests.

These chemicals, over years of use, leach into the soil and the water supply and become part of the physiology of the people around these communities.

Many pesticides have now been banned for use because of their detrimental effects on human physiology. DDT, DDE and many others have been banned worldwide because they are both carcinogenic and neurotoxic. Again we have to ask the question—why they weren't tested earlier?

TOXIC BURDEN

To become better educated about detoxification, a little terminology is important. We'll need to understand what we mean by *exogenous* and *endogenous* toxins and more importantly how we define a word we've often used, *body burden*.

Chemical toxins are divided into two groups, exogenous and endogenous. Exogenous toxins are present in the outside environment. These are found in the air we breathe, the water we drink, the food we consume, and the things we apply to our skin. Endogenous toxins are those produced within the body from various metabolic activities including the activity of micro-organisms found in the gastrointestinal tract. The body has detoxification mechanisms to deal with these kinds of toxic substances, but when high levels of toxins overwhelm physiological tolerance, problems will arise.

To describe how much toxicity is in the body at any given time you'll often hear the term *body burden* being used. The problem with this term is that we really don't know exactly how many chemicals are present, so even though the term serves a purpose, it has its limitations. Yet, it can be useful, especially when talking about how to reduce overall toxic accumulation.

The only way of reducing overall body burden is to first reduce your total exposure and then enhance your body's ability to detoxify. What we need to learn is where our exposure comes from so we can begin the process of reducing this exposure. For example, you have learned that most foods carry pesticide residue. One of the ways you can reduce this exposure is to consume organic foods.

TOXIC BURDEN = Total Amount of Toxins Consumed – Ability of the Body to Detoxify

There have been recent arguments about whether or not organic foods are more nutritious for you. But the primary purpose of eating organic food is to reduce the agricultural chemicals you are exposed to when you eat conventionally-grown produce.. Certified organic foods are free of pesticides, herbicides, and other chemicals you should avoid.

The second way of reducing your body burden is to improve the body's ability to eliminate toxins. This revolves around enhancing the detoxification systems in the body, including the Phase I and II systems in the liver. Along the same lines, we want to improve the elimination process through the digestive tract. By enhancing these systems, our ability to get rid of toxins will also improve. The end result should be a reduced body burden. Let's take a closer look at toxic metals.

THE MOST COMMON ENVIRONMENTAL TOXINS

Toxic metals, which are sometimes referred to as heavy metals, have become so prominent in the environment that most of us know their names. They include mercury, lead, cadmium, aluminum, and arsenic. Some scientists believe that toxic metals are the more dangerous than other organic substances such as pesticides and herbicides.

Toxic metals make their way into our physiology through a number of different channels. They can be inhaled as fumes or dust particles. We can also ingest them through the food we eat and the water we drink. Another way metals can enter our body is through the skin—for example aluminum-based antiperspirants or lipsticks containing lead.

In the end there is little doubt that toxic metals are finding their way into our bodies, where they affect our physiology. One area of grave concern is toxic metals' ability to inhibit the activity of various enzyme systems throughout the body. Enzymes are mostly proteins that make everything in your body work. The scientific definition of enzymes is that they are bio-molecules that increase the rate of chemical reactions. In other words, enzymes speed things up and without them, reactions essential for life would not be possible.

Enzymes allow you to digest foods. Without them, foods would sit in your gut and basically rot. Enzymes allow you to make hormones and other important chemicals our bodies need. They also help to create the energy molecule ATP. It is safe to say that enzymes are essential for every single reaction in the body—enzymes are essential for life.

When contaminants such as toxic metals can affect the activity of enzymes, the amount of enzymes inhibited and the degree of inhibition depends on how serious the toxicity is. Toxic metals can affect a broad range of enzymes and, depending on the body burden, can have anywhere from mild symptom patterns to serious. If the body burden is extreme, toxic metal poisoning can even cause death.

There is little doubt that toxic metals are accumulating in the body's organs. Once the organ accumulates high levels of these toxic metals, symptoms result. Organs involved can include the liver, kidneys, gastrointestinal tract, and even the brain. Here are some of the most common metals to watch for:

LEAD: Although new legislation has removed lead from paint and gasoline, exposure is still a public health concern in the United States. There are still approximately 21 million homes with lead-based paint on their walls. Flaking, weathering, and chalking paint contaminate dust and soil, contributing to lead exposure. Lead is also used in battery manufacturing, the printing industry, firing ranges, the plastic industry, and the rubber industry. And, as we've seen with lipstick, lead is even in the cosmetic industry.

Water from old leaded pipes, soldered plumbing, and water cooling systems are additional sources of lead. If you have leaded pipes in your building, you could be exposing yourself, especially in the morning when water has been in contact with the pipes all night. Make sure you run the water in the morning for a period of time before consuming it.

As I've already mentioned, lead is a known toxin affecting the nervous system. It causes learning and behavioral problems. Studies show that lead lowers IQ, reduces school performance, and increases aggression. Expectant mothers need to be aware of this because lead easily crosses the placenta and may affect the fetal brain where it can interfere with normal development. Lead has also been linked to miscarriages and reduced fertility.

Lead competes in the body with calcium, causing numerous malfunctions in calcium-facilitated cellular mechanisms. When you think about this aspect alone, you can see the vast consequences that could result. Calcium is important for bone health, heart function, muscle movement, and many other important processes. Impeding its action can lead to serious problems.

The central nervous system (CNS) appears to be most affected by lead. Children in particular are susceptible to its devastating effects on mental development and intelligence. Cerebro-behavioral deficits, such as attention deficit disorder, have also been found in lead-exposed children. Blood lead concentrations of 20-25 µg/100 ml can cause irreversible CNS damage in children.

Acute lead exposure in adults often affects the kidneys. Chronic exposure, however, can cause kidney dysfunction characterized by high blood pressure, high uric acid levels (leading to gout), and kidney failure.

After lead is absorbed, the human body tries to use its natural antioxidants such as glutathione to eliminate it. Unfortunately, this causes liver glutathione to be depleted very quickly, resulting in less glutathione being available for other detoxification reactions. This leads to a vicious cycle of impaired detoxification mechanisms which increases systemic chemical toxins.

MERCURY: This is a well known toxic metal that has become a major concern. Humans are exposed to mercury primarily in two forms: mercury vapor and methyl mercury compounds. Both of these forms are absorbed through the lungs and digestive tract respectively, eventually making their way into the nervous system where mercury does most of its damage.

To gain a better understanding of this toxic metal, it's helpful to have a little background on the different forms of mercury. Elemental mercury is what is used in thermometers, switching devices, vacuum pumps, pressure sensing devices, and the amalgams fillings used in dental offices. Elemental mercury, or metallic mercury as it is also called, is poorly absorbed by the digestive tract. However, touching this type of mercury is very dangerous since it is easily absorbed through the skin.

Elemental mercury is also the type of mercury that is spewed into the environment from power plants that burn coal, as well as waste incinerators, paper processing factories, and smelting operations. Mercury from these sources is released into the air and is eventually deposited into oceans and other water ways in the form of rain.

Once in the ocean, it settles to the bottom where bacteria and other microorganisms convert it to methyl mercury. Fish absorb this methyl mercury thorough their gills and by consuming food sources that contain it. Mercury then binds to proteins that make up the muscle tissue.

This is why a large numbers of predatory fish now contain high levels of mercury. In fact according to the EPA there was a 163 percent increase in fish mercury levels from 1993 to 2003.

In my own practice, I see a direct correlation between dietary fish intake and mercury levels in the blood. Living on the West Coast, many of my patients consume high levels of sushi including tuna, a predatory fish usually contaminated with high levels of mercury. During routine toxic metal testing I find elevated mercury levels in a majority of the cases.

Interestingly enough, an article appearing in the *New York Times* on January 23, 2008 confirms the problem with tuna. The *New York Times*, through an independent lab, analyzed the mercury content of tuna served in 20 sushi restaurants. They found that five of them had mercury levels so high that the FDA (Food and Drug Administration) could have taken legal action to remove the fish from the market.

Once contaminated tuna is ingested, over 90 percent of the methyl mercury from the fish is absorbed into the blood stream. Studies show that, in pregnant women, this mercury can cross the placenta and accumulate in the developing fetus. Methyl mercury can also find its way into breast milk. The problem has gotten so bad that physicians are now warning pregnant women and breast feeding moms about the dangers of methyl mercury.

Once inside the cells of the body, mercury can cause a number of symptoms. The symptoms and damage caused depend on how much has entered the body, the amount of time the body is exposed, and how well the body detoxifies it. Its primary physiological targets are the central nervous system, including the brain, as well as the endocrine system, kidneys, and other organs. Some of the symptoms include impairment of peripheral vision, skin discoloration, disturbances in sensations (pins and needles, numbness in the feet and around the mouth), lack of coordination, impaired speech and hearing, muscle weakness, desquamation (dead skin peels off in layers), mood swings, memory loss, and mental disturbances.

When the developing fetus and young children come in contact with high levels of mercury, their brains can sustain damage that will eventually affect the way they think and their ability to learn. Mercury is a very serious problem and we need to become better educated on how to reduce our own exposure and that of our children.

Fish is not the only way we encounter mercury. Mercury-based dental fillings are the major source of inorganic mercury exposure in humans. Most scientists agree that mercury amalgam fillings (mercury amalgam means an alloy of mercury and other metals), expose people with these fillings to a daily dose of mercury. The debate is centered on the levels that are released. Some argue that the levels are too low to cause any real damage while others counter those arguments with evidence claiming that long- term build up will eventually cause harm.

Even as mercury amalgams are prepared and placed in the patient's mouth, the dentist, dental assistant, and the patient, are exposed to mercury vapor (HgO). This vapor enters the blood stream after being inhaled into the lungs. The patient is further exposed to mercury vapor as the amalgam releases HgO whenever the individual chews, brushes or drinks hot beverages. Studies of mercury content in the exhaled breath of those with and without amalgams have found significantly higher baseline mercury levels in subjects with amalgams—and up to a 15-fold increase in mercury in expired air after chewing. Mercury release was found to be greater in old corroded amalgams compared to new, polished ones.

In humans, 90 percent of mercury elimination is via the feces in association with glutathione, with only 10 percent normally being excreted in the urine. A decrease in hepatic glutathione resulting from mercury excretion can compromise other liver functions that are dependent upon glutathione for detoxification. One thing we should be learn from this is that glutathione is important in detoxification and we should do everything we can to increase its levels.

CADMIUM: Environmental cadmium exposure comes from a variety of sources. For example, dust from automobile tires as they erode, incinerators burning waste, fertilizers, rechargeable batteries, coffee, and cigarette smoke. In fact, smokers have four to five times higher blood levels of cadmium and two to three time's higher cadmium concentrations in their kidneys.

Cadmium, as well as lead and mercury, can interact metabolically with nutritionally essential metals. Cadmium interacts with calcium in the skeletal system to produce osteodystrophies (defective bone development). It also competes with zinc for binding sites on specific proteins called metallothionein, which is important in the storage and transport of zinc during development. But it doesn't stop there. Cadmium can actually replace zinc in many biological systems because it can bind 10 times more strongly than zinc. This causes many problems since zinc takes part in over 200 enzymatic reactions that carry out important physiological functions.

When cadmium reaches threshold levels, damage to the kidney may occur. Biliary excretion seems to be an essential factor for the fecal elimination of cadmium, although this metal may be also excreted in the urine.

PESTICIDES

As mentioned previously, pesticides are another major contaminant that can affect human health. They are a particular threat because they are found in about up to 90 percent of the foods we eat. That's right, most of the foods you consume—unless they are certified organic—contain pesticide residue. Fresh fruits and vegetables, cereals, breads, beverages, and even coffee contain these toxic chemicals.

Pesticides are synthetic chemicals that control insects, rodents, and other organisms that we consider to be pests. These chemicals are obviously toxic since their primary purpose is to kill living things. Why we would assume that these chemicals would have no effect on humans?

The American Medical Association recommends limits on our exposure to pesticides because of their possible negative effects. One concern is the long-term effect of low dose pesticide exposure. There are studies that link pesticide exposure to long-term health problems including memory disorders, dermatologic conditions, cancers, depression, neurological problems, miscarriages, and birth defects. Based on this evidence, we should limit our exposure.

There have been many studies of farmers with the goal of determining the health effects of pesticide exposure. But many farmers already have the evidence they need. Even in my wife's family, you can easily see the effects long term pesticide use can have. As mentioned earlier my wife's father died of bladder cancer at the age of 42, her mother has fibromyalgia, her sister has endocrine issues, and her brother has rheumatoid arthritis at 27 years of age. This is not coincidence; it is from chemical exposure.

The World Health Organization estimates that each year three million agricultural workers in the developing world experience severe poisoning from pesticides; of those, about 18,000 die. In one study, the researchers estimate that as many as 25 million workers in developing countries suffer mild pesticide poisoning yearly. Other research carried out by the National Institute of Health has linked pesticide exposure to diabetes. A paper published in the *American Journal of Epidemiology* concluded that the association between specific pesticides and the incidence of diabetes ranged from a 30 to 200 percent increase in risk.

About 90 percent of all pesticide use in the United States is in agriculture. However, more than 80 percent of these pesticides reach a destination other than their intended target. They instead end up in non-targeted water ways, air, soil, and food. Pesticides can be carried by the wind to other areas, contaminating them as well. They can add to water pollution, soil contamination, and can be classified as persistent organic pollutants. Yet, agriculture is not the only industry utilizing these toxic chemicals. Pesticides are used in paints, carpets, shampoos, hair wigs, disposal diapers, and contact lenses. Many pet products like flea collars and pet shampoos also contain pesticides. These toxins eventually find their way into carpeting, bedding, and even food.

There are a number of different categories of pesticides; the main three include organophosphates, organochlorine and carbamates.

ORGANOPHOSPHATES: These pesticides were originally developed as chemical warfare agents. However, because they seem to be less damaging to the environment and less persistent than other types of pesticides, their use has increased. This does not make them safe for humans. As a matter of fact, organophosphates have poisoned more people then other types of pesticides.

These pesticides are readily absorbed through the skin, lungs, and digestive tract. Most people that have toxicity are directly exposed to organophosphate during their application (crop spraying). Since most of these chemicals affect the nervous system, including the brain, toxicity symptoms are numerous. For example, some symptoms include dizziness, abdominal pain, headaches, nausea, and vomiting as well as skin and eye problems.

ORGANOCHLORINES: Organochlorines are used specifically to control insects, unlike other pesticides that can also destroy rodents. These pesticides are well absorbed and accumulate easily in fatty tissues around the body. For example, a study appearing in *Toxicology Sciences* demonstrated that when obese subjects go on calorie restricted diets and begin to lose fat, organochloride pesticide levels rise. This study, published in 2002, also showed that the elevated blood levels disrupted thyroid hormone production. Organochlorides can also be carcinogenic and can affect the central nervous system including the brain. Symptoms can include dizziness, nausea, tremors, headaches, slurred speech, and poor balance.

Perhaps the best known organochloride is the banned pesticide DDT (dichlorodiphenyltrichloroethane). DDT was banned in the 1970's because of its effects on the environment. But DDT has an interesting history that began during World War II when it became popular as a pesticide for controlling mosquitoes transmitting malaria and lice. It wasn't till Rachel Carson's *Silent Spring* hit the bookstands in 1962 that DDT became a target. She suggested that this pesticide could cause cancer and that it was having a detrimental effect on wildlife. Subsequent research proved that she was right and DDT became a public enemy.

Even though DDT has been banned for more than 30 years, its persistence in the environment continues. A by-product of DDT, known as DDE, has also been linked to women who have breast cancer. It seems that women who develop breast cancer have higher residues of DDE in their breasts than do those that do not have the disease.

CARBAMATES: The advantage of carbamate pesticides is that they are more biodegradable than organophosphates. They are very widely used for their fungicidal and herbicidal properties. Unlike other pesticides, they do not bioaccumulate in mammals but they do concentrate in fish. Some of these carbamates can cause liver and kidney problems.

TOXINS AROUND YOUR HOUSE

If we are going to reduce our overall exposure to chemical toxins we obviously need to learn about them—especially where they are coming from. Thus far, we've discussed some major players in the toxic world, including pesticides and toxic metals. In this section we are going to focus on toxins that are very close to you—the ones that actually live with you in your own home.

We think of our homes as havens, places where we relax, have our meals, sleep, and play with our kids; our private shelter from the outside world. Yet, there are more toxins floating around inside your home than all of the pollutants outside of it. In fact, the inside of a home can be 25 to 100 times more toxic than the outside environment.

When you begin to evaluate the household items, building materials, and cleaning products used in the home, you'll begin to discover an incredible array of chemicals that contribute to our overall exposure. Homes can, in fact, be so toxic that you can develop sick building syndrome. We discussed this disease earlier, yet the mere fact that medical science has actually acknowledge it gives you an idea of how powerful these chemical toxins can be. Yet, most people don't understand the seriousness of the problem.

In a survey conducted by the Environmental Protection Agency (EPA), 95 percent of moms agreed that household cleaning products can be toxic, but only 49 percent thought that their kids could be exposed to them. What's more, only 33 percent of consumers surveyed agreed that indoor air is more toxic then outdoor. So people know that there are chemicals but not everyone understands that they are causing harm to their own bodies and possibly their children.

According to the EPA, the average American home generates about 20 pounds of hazardous waste every year. That translates to about 3.2 billion pounds of household hazardous waster per year—176,000 tons just from cleaning products. This includes tile, toilet, kitchen, floor, and oven cleaners. There are also solvents and formaldehyde (found in drapes and carpets), phenol (cleaning products), toluene (glues, correction fluids), benzene (dyes, insecticides), wood preservatives, 1,4 dicholorobenzene (disinfectants), and volatile organic compounds. There are even foods that can create chemicals that impact your physiology. For example, microwave popcorn contains chemicals that stop the liquid oils from seeping through the bag. The chemical formed as the kernels pop is perfluorooctanoic acid (PFOA). This chemical my cause birth defects, reduce baby's birth weight, and is possibly be linked to cancer.

Of course, there are many more examples, but the point is this: It's time to clean things up—and, like charity, it should begin at home.

REDUCING BODY BURDEN

There is little doubt about the fact that chemical toxins, including toxic metals, are getting into our bodies. They have infiltrated more than just our environment. Identifying these substances and their sources is the first step in reducing overall exposure. Once you identify key toxic compounds, you can become better equipped to avoid them and thus reduce your overall body burden.

4

Health Effects of Toxins

YOU HAVE PROBABLY HEARD IT SAID that we are what we drink, eat, breathe, touch, and can't eliminate. Forty years ago this would have been ignored by many, but today there is an impressive body of scientific evidence that supports this very notion. Research is pointing to the fact that environmental toxins, including the food we eat and the water we drink, are having a serious impact on our health. We are discovering that pesticides are causing cancer and that various types of plastic additives are influencing and changing the hormone levels in our bodies.

Some evidence suggests that there may be a link between autism and mercury through vaccinations, although this topic is still quite controversial. Other studies suggest that childhood cancers may be related to the enormous number of chemical toxins we are exposed to. Even things we don't consider toxic take a toll on our bodies. For example, the average American consumes over 150 pounds of refined sugar each year. This not only puts them at risk for diabetes, but it increases the odds of heart disease, autoimmune problems, and nervous system disorders.

WHAT ABOUT THE LIVER?

Doesn't the body get rid of toxins through the liver? While it's true that the body gets rid of chemicals primarily through the liver, the body also detoxifies itself through a number of other organ systems. What's more, the liver is designed to filter natural toxicities in a natural environment—not the synthetic toxins that now infiltrate every aspect of our lives.

There are many toxic substances created through normal metabolic functions. For example, one of the by-products when we breathe in oxygen is carbon dioxide. Carbon dioxide can be toxic at high levels; however, our lungs naturally remove it from our bodies when we exhale. This is natural and the body can easily handle this load. There are numerous other examples, like protein metabolism and sugar metabolism which also creates toxic chemicals that the body naturally detoxifies.

But when we put things into our body that don't occur in nature, the body has to go through more complex mechanisms to get rid of them. This isn't normally a problem, but high levels of toxins can cause difficulties. An example of this is alcohol consumption. Having one drink is tolerable and you will feel fine. Your liver will rapidly detoxify the alcohol and your blood levels will be under the legal limit. But if you drink a bottle of vodka, it's a whole different story. You will become intoxicated and may experience dizziness, slurred speech, imbalance, upset stomach, and the next day, a hangover. So what happened to your detoxification system? The toxic load (the amount of alcohol consumed) was higher than your body's ability to detoxify.

HIPPOCRATES SEEMED TO KNOW

In 500 B.C., Hippocrates, the "father of medicine," proclaimed that we should look for disease in the environment around us—in the food we eat, the water we drink, and the air we breathe. Nearly 2,500 years later, after thousands of medical breakthroughs and discoveries, it seems that Hippocrates had it right from the beginning. He and other ancient physicians knew that the body had to be in harmony—not only within itself, but with the environment that surrounded it.

Today more than ever, science is beginning to realize that it is indeed the environment around us that may be responsible for what is happening within us. That the things we are putting in our bodies, the things we come in contact with, are creating such an imbalance that disease is the end result. We are also learning that moving away from the natural environment by changing it will also change our internal environment. This will ultimately change us.

OUR BIOLOGICAL ENVIRONMENT

One of the biggest problems in modern medicine is its stubborn obsession with symptoms. When you go see your family physician for a specific problem, your diagnoses results from what best fits your symptoms based on your medical history and possible testing procedures. You will be given a name for your problem and then most likely a medication of some sort, either over-the-counter or prescription. Here is a typical example of their thinking: Your ulcer is painful because stomach acid is coming in contact with the lining of your stomach, so let's just remove the acid.

This concept of treating the symptoms does not address what the causative factor or factors of the ulcer actually are. This approach will lead to an alkalinization of the stomach and duodenum that will reduce the ulcer symptoms but create a number of digestive problems that, long term, can lead to serious chronic disease health issues.

But when you look at the symptoms as a part of the whole body, responsive to events in the body's environment, then you are on the path to healing. For example, when somebody has an ulcer, all systems are checked and a history is completed to find out the cause of the ulcer (i.e., stress, non-steroidal anti-inflammatories or diet). Once the cause is uncovered, it is addressed and, at the same time, measures are taken to improve the health of the mucosal lining causing the ulcer symptoms. This is done without changing the acidity but instead by helping the body heal the ulceration with proper nutrition.

This approach to medicine takes care of the biological environment. Remember, the body is in a constant battle to keep homeostasis (be in balance). For example, we need a certain amount of calcium floating around the blood stream at all times. When calcium levels are low, the body releases certain hormones (specifically, parathyroid hormone) to loosen calcium from bones in order to bring calcium to the right biological level. If, on the other hand, you have too much circulating calcium, the body sends out other hormones (calcitonin) in order to store calcium and reduce circulating levels. There are numerous other examples of this that take place within other systems in the body. A change in the environment—internally and externally—will trigger a number of events that will alter various body systems.

GENETICS MAY NOT BE DESTINY

To shed some light into what may be going on within the various systems of the body, let's once again review the fascinating article about the twins that appeared in *Discover* magazine (November 2006). The article indirectly outlined the impact that the environment can have on the human body. In the beginning of the article, a scientific picture of two distinctly different individuals appeared (see figure 4.1). One individual is obviously taller and larger than the other and they both appear to have different facial features. At first glance, that's basically all the observational analysis one can do, but further digging reveals something very interesting. What it discloses is nothing short of shocking—that these two individuals are in fact identical twins. Now identical twins are supposed to be indistinguishable yet these two are far from the same. What happened? When scientists studied this anomaly they discovered something quite remarkable. They found that these individuals had been separated at birth and grew up in two very different environments. The foods they consumed, the water they drank, the air they breathed, and the nurturing they received was different—and it was that difference that changed the behavior of their DNA.

Titled "DNA Is Not Destiny," the article reviewed how the environment can effect how DNA is actually read by the body. What this may eventually prove is the reasons we develop cancer or get heart disease is not because we inherit them from our parents, but rather because we do exactly what our parents did. The moral of the story is that the things we are exposed to will, in the end, be responsible for not only the diseases we may acquire but also the way we look.

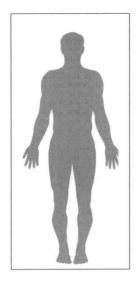 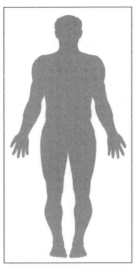

FIGURE 3.1: *Discovery* magazine: **Identical** twins separated at birth

The article discusses how different foods have a dramatic effect on the expression of the DNA. This can impact both your health and the way you look.

SOME BACKGROUND

This is nothing new. As I mentioned, Hippocrates directed us to, to look at the environment to find the cause of disease. This insight is only now just being realized by the scientific community. There have been pioneers in this area of study for decades but we have not been listening.

Knowledge of toxic chemicals and their negative effect on human health and wildlife populations were discussed as far back as the 1960's when Rachel Carson's *Silent Spring* became the candle glowing in the darkness. The book shed light on the tremendous number of toxins being dumped into the environment and the potential long-term effects. Carson believed that a day would come when the spring would be silent because most wildlife would have been destroyed by the environmental poisons around them.

Scientists began suspecting that man-made chemicals interfered with hormones around the same time Carson's book was published. Since then, there has been much published on toxic chemicals and their impact on the wildlife populations. Studies in the Great Lakes region have shown both fish and bird populations effected by the high levels of toxins polluting these immense waterways. In ponds across the Midwest, male frogs began laying eggs after exposure to the herbicide atrazine.

According to an article in the *Dallas News* which appeared in May, 2007, more than 200 scientists signed a declaration warning that exposure to chemicals in the womb may make babies more likely to develop diabetes, obesity, attention deficit disorder, and infertility. They recognized that our environment is in crisis and action needs to be taken to halt the serious health risks it may cause.

WHAT CAN THESE CHEMICALS DO?

Chemicals can enter the body through the skin, the digestive system, and the respiratory tract. Once inside your body, these toxins can cause untold harm. They can interfere with the synthesis of certain important molecules like hormones, neurotransmitters, and immune communicating cells. These chemicals can even have effects on structural entities like the mitochondria of cells which are critical in energy production. Although there are some conflicting studies, it is safe to assume that toxins are in no way beneficial to health. Logic alone tells us that these synthetic chemicals are detrimental to the human body.

One way that we see how toxic chemicals might damage the human body is through the animal model. Researchers use animals to begin the rigorous process of studying medicines for eventual use in humans. For example, when researchers begin doing studies on a possible cancer drug, they first try the drug on animal models. In order to do so they have to give the animals cancer. How do you suppose they do that? They expose them the chemical toxin DMBA (dimethylbenzanthracene). This induces biochemical changes that create cancer.

We can draw similar parallels when it comes to the environmental toxins that humans are constantly being exposed to. If chemical toxins induce cancer in animals models, aren't they capable of doing the same thing in humans? Scientists are definitely starting to buy into this theory and are beginning to be more vocal when it comes to expressing these views.

Ana Soto, M.D., professor of anatomy and cellular biology at Tufts University School of Medicine, states that, in the 1940's, a woman's risk of breast cancer was one in 22. Today the risk has risen to one in eight. Genetics is only a cause in about 5 to 10 percent of the cases yet this is where most research is focused. According to Soto, it is time to focus our efforts on environmental toxins, since the increasing risk of breast and other cancers has paralleled the proliferation of synthetic chemicals introduced since World War II. This again brings us back to the story of the twins, where these individuals had the exact same genes yet they became two very different people. Their genes didn't cause these differences; it was instead their exposure to environmental triggers.

In a medical review appearing in the *Journal of the National Cancer Institute*, the author states that cancer incidence could be reduced as much as 90 percent just with the elimination of environmental toxins. A *British Medical Journal* review touts that nearly 75 percent of most cancer are environmentally induced. And cancer is just one of many illnesses associated with environmental chemicals. Toxins have also been linked to autoimmune diseases, neurological problems, and endocrine disorders including the thyroid, adrenal, and reproductive glands.

These kinds of statements from legitimate researchers and publications are just part of the movement that is finally beginning to acknowledge the contentions Rachel Carson made nearly half a century ago. We are now not looking at whether or not the environment is having an impact, but specifically how it affects human health—and what can be done to stop it. There has been a shift. It is a shift in the right direction, but we must continue to apply pressure for the changes we need to have a viable future on this planet.

One of the ways toxins can lead to cancer is because they can have a profoundly negative effect of the proper function of the immune system, our first line of defense against many cancers.

IMMUNE SYSTEM

Environmental toxins can also have wide-ranging effects on the immune system. They can weaken immunity, causing increased susceptibility to infections and cancer. Toxins can also make the immune system overly sensitive, giving rise to allergies and autoimmune disease.

Research has shown that chlorinated pesticides, polycyclic hydrocarbons (PAHs), and organophosphate pesticides all have toxic effects on the immune system.

An area of environmental medicine that always gets lots of press is heavy metals and their effects on the nervous system. Since the nervous system requires the action of a complex integrated network (like a circuit board), damage to even a small section of the system can have serious consequences. For example, research shows that exposure to lead in children and animals living around industrial environments produce behavioral impairment.

Aluminum is another metal of concern. People with high concentration of aluminum in nerve tissue have a higher incidence of Alzheimer's disease and dementia. The aluminum comes from the water supply, food, antacids, and antiperspirants.

Knowing how aluminum works in deodorants and antiperspirants is insightful in understanding its neurotoxic capabilities. Aluminum is used in these products because after application it can make its way into cells, swelling them and plugging up the ability of the duct to allow sweat to exit. Several animal studies have established that aluminum is a neurotoxin, meaning toxic to the brain. Its negative effects on the brain are well known and it is capable of causing DNA damage and can have adverse epigenetic effects as well.

A CLOSER LOOK

In this section, we will take a closer look at what common toxins are doing to the body. The first part will look at general, non-specific damage that can lead to many systemic problems. Some of these you'll recognize, others will be new. The idea is to get a grasp of the ongoing assault your body is constantly under and its struggle to keep things in balance.

In the second part, we will explore specific health conditions and how chemical toxins are contributing to their spread. Here we are trying to again link the chronic diseases of this century with chemical toxins. I will provide the evidence that may explain why these diseases are so prevalent and why modern medicine has had such a hard time solving them.

THE MICRO EFFECTS OF TOXINS

Usually what happens on the micro (invisible to the human eye) level will eventually be experienced on a macro (visible to the eye) one. So having some idea of what is going on molecularly has importance in understanding the effects of toxins.

Most of my patients have heard the term *free radical damage*, but they usually don't know what it really means. They know that refined sugar is not healthy, but they never relate it to a process known as glycation. These might sound like complicated terms, but when we break them down, we find that they are actually simple concepts. Understanding these concepts will give us a greater appreciation of why we need to minimize toxic exposure and support our body's own detoxification systems.

FREE RADICAL DAMAGE

Most people have heard the term *antioxidant* and some of those same people have heard the more complicated term *free radical*. In reality, both terms are used often but few really have a grasp about their meaning and the big role they play in pathologies, including aging.

In science, free radicals are atoms or group of atoms (organic molecules) containing unpaired electrons. In nature, electrons want to be paired. A free radical is unpaired and wants another electron so it can become stable. Once this free radical steals an electron from another atom, that atom then becomes a free radical. This process begins a chain reaction that can damage cells in the body. A good analogy of free radical damage is rust, an oxidation process that leads to damage on metal surfaces.

Another example I often use to explain free radicals and antioxidants is the apple and lemon juice analogy. If you take an apple and slice it in half, the white flesh will quickly begin to brown. This browning is caused by free radical damage. A free radical begins stealing an electron from the apple cells which cause a chain reaction creating the browning effect. But if you had placed lemon juice on half that apple, it would have acted like an antioxidant and prevented the apple from browning (Fig 4.1).

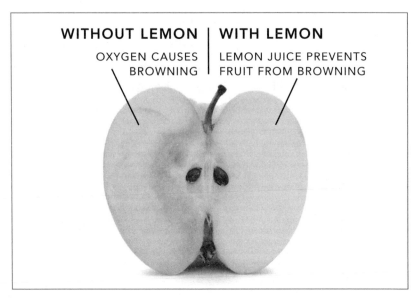

WITHOUT LEMON | **WITH LEMON**

OXYGEN CAUSES | LEMON JUICE PREVENTS
BROWNING | FRUIT FROM BROWNING

FIGURE 4.1 Browning of apple and the antioxidant effects of lemon juice.

Antioxidants provide the electron that the free radical is missing. Once that electron is replaced, everything is back to normal. From this simple understanding, you can expand it to virtually all biochemical processes in the body that are at risk of free radical damage.

Free radicals also have a purpose. They are made in the body through a vast number of ongoing metabolic processes. For example, because free radicals are so damaging, they are produced within certain types of white blood cells to kill viruses and bacteria. In other words free radicals play an important role in boosting your immune system activity.

Free radicals are also produced from all sorts of other biochemical processes like energy production in mitochondria (energy factories in cells), detoxification processes, synthesis of inflammatory compounds, and a host of other reactions. All and all we have free radicals being produced through normal body metabolic processes.

Unfortunately, toxins can create a high load of free radicals. As I've just mentioned, free radicals are naturally produced in the body and, under normal environmental conditions, the body neutralizes them. However, in today's toxic world, the body's environment is far from normal. There is an excess of free radical proliferation caused by a numbers of environmental pollutants and lifestyles.

Excess proliferation of free radicals comes from:

- Hydrocarbons from residuals of cigarette smoke.
- Toxic metals.
- Chlorinated hydrocarbons.
- Rancid fats.
- Reduction in the supply of oxygen to they body's organs because of a sedentary lifestyle.
- Stress.

Take note that much of the free radical load in the body is attributable to the massive influx of toxic chemicals. These chemicals are creating the overload of circulating free radicals, creating an enormous burden on the body's antioxidant reserves. Studies have verified that, compared to unexposed people, Vitamin C (antioxidant) blood levels were significantly lower in smokers, alcoholics, and people exposed to higher levels of toxins.

When we have a proliferation of free radicals we can experience extensive damage to our DNA, proteins, and fats, which can contribute to or cause dozens of different acute and chronic diseases. The most notable of these diseases are atherosclerosis, angina, stroke, congestive heart failure, cancer, metabolic syndrome, diabetes, pregnancy toxemia, allergies, asthma, Parkinson's disease, and aging.

Free radicals attack DNA and almost every cellular component in the body, which means they can have a vast array of negative consequence on human health. Getting them under control by reducing exposure and increasing antioxidant reserves is very important.

GLYCATION

A real problem with the way we eat is the tremendous amount of sugar we consume. The average American consumes approximately 150 pounds of refined sugar (sucrose) every year and about 50 pounds of high fructose corn syrup. In total we are consuming in excess of 200 pounds of sugar annually. That's a tremendous amount. Our body was made to consume complex carbohydrates that eventually breakdown to the simple sugars needed for energy production. It was not made to process refined sugar that greatly increases blood sugar and triggers huge releases of insulin.

When sugar enters the blood stream, it needs to make its way inside the cells where it can be utilized as energy. This is accomplished with insulin. But this incredible hormone was not made to handle the tremendous load of refined carbohydrate that it now faces daily. Your blood stream has a huge amount of sugar coming into it, so it needs to call on insulin often. This elevation and high usage of insulin creates problems on cell surfaces, where insulin works. The cells become less sensitive to insulin and this results in us consuming even more sugar.

The end result is more than just susceptibility to diabetes. We are all aware of the fact that a diet high in sugar is associated with Type II diabetes. But did you know that all of that sugar creates high blood sugar levels which lead to a process called glycation? Glycation is a term used to describe the process that occurs when sugar binds to proteins or fats in the blood stream randomly, without any controlling mechanisms. The end result of this process is the impaired functioning of many bio-molecules that may include enzymes, hormones, and neurotransmitters.

To get a better idea of how this happens, let me give you the "can of pop" analogy. When you open a can of pop and leave out for a day, what do you feel when you pick it up? It feels sticky. That's because sugar acts like glue and can bind to lots of things it comes in contact with.

When sugar is circulating in the blood stream, it can easily go through glycation. The first steps of advanced glycation are slow reactions that create a number of end products called glycation end products (AGE's). Some AGE's are neutral but others can be very reactive and have been linked to a number of serious chronic conditions that include Type I and II diabetes, heart disease, Alzheimer's disease, cancer, peripheral neuropathy, and a number of other conditions. The message here is that sugar is a toxin and works on the micro level, giving rise to a number of chronic diseases.

HEALTH EFFECTS OF EXPOSURE TO CHEMICAL TOXINS

If there is one thing we should be starting to realize, it's how vulnerable we actually are to toxic chemicals. They are everywhere, even in places we thought sacred. For example, did you ever think that sugar could have such broad toxic effects on your body? The reality is that it does, and it's only one of the thousands of ingredients that are attacking our bodies and causing possible harm.

To get a better idea of what specific systems these chemicals attack, we are going to go through four main areas of concern—endocrine disruptors, neurotoxins, immune system suppressants, and carcinogens. These are systems that the scientific community has gathered enough evidence on to show that something needs to be done. When chemicals are affecting our hormones, nerve conduction pathways, and immune function, while increasing our risk for a variety of cancers, we need to be concerned.

ENDOCRINE DISRUPTORS

The endocrine system is a network of glands and hormones that regulate many of the body's functions. They include growth and development, regulation of organ systems, and most of the biological systems in the body. For example, these hormones communicate with the body, bringing about changes in metabolism, repair mechanisms, sexual reproduction, and digestion.

The glands that make up the endocrine system include the pineal, pituitary, thyroid, thymus, pancreas, ovaries, and testes. These glands release carefully-measured amounts of hormones into the bloodstream that act as natural chemical messengers, traveling to different parts of the body in order to control and adjust many biological functions. It is safe to say that the endocrine system is a critical component of the physiological functioning of the human body. Knowing that the hormones this system make and release are so carefully controlled and, on a relative scale, are produced in very minute amounts, disrupting this system can have numerous negative consequences on general health.

Endocrine disruptors are synthetic chemicals that, once inside the body, can either mimic or block hormones and thus disrupt the body's normal endocrine function. This can happen through a number of different mechanisms:

- By reducing the production of the hormone in the endocrine gland.
- By affecting the release of the hormone from the gland.
- By mimicking or counteracting the effect of the hormone at the sight it is suppose to effect.
- By speeding up the breakdown of the hormone, therefore reducing is activity.

Let's see how this would look if the hormone involved was insulin. If the endocrine disruptor were to counteract the effect of insulin, it would go to the sight insulin is suppose to affect (the cell) and block it from actually doing its job. Since insulin's job is to shuttle sugar into the cell, this would not occur and we would have elevated blood sugar level.

Chemicals that are known human endocrine disruptors include diethylstilbesterol (the drug DES), dioxins, plasticizers like BPA and phthalates, PCBs, and DDT. Many chemicals, particularly pesticides and plasticizers, are suspected endocrine disruptors based on limited animal studies.

THE EVIDENCE OF THEIR DANGERS

There is a growing body of evidence-based toxicology studies, wildlife studies, and epidemiology suggesting that endocrine disruptors are a threat to human health. For example, fish in the Great Lakes that are contaminated with PCBs and other man-made chemicals have numerous reproductive problems, as well as abnormal swelling of the thyroid gland. In the same area, fish-eating birds such as eagles, terns, and gulls were shown to have similar dysfunctions. Scientists have also pointed

TABLE 4.1

Endocrine Disruptors	What They Are	Sources
PCBs (polychlorinated biphenyls)	Non-flammable, stable synthetic compounds that exhibit electrical insulating properties.	Used in coolants, lubricants in transformers, and other electrical equipment
DDT (dichloro-diphenyl-trichloroethane)	Colorless odorless pesticide used in the 1950's to destroy disease carrying insects. Banned in 1970's.	Agricultural chemical persistent in the environment and in the food chain.
Dioxins (chlorinated organic chemicals)	Group of chlorinated organic chemicals.	Formed as by-products of human activities such as waste incineration, fuel combustion, chlorine bleaching of pulp and paper.
DES (diethyl-stilbestrol)	Orally active synthetic non-steroidal estrogen used to prevent miscarriages in the 1950's. Found to be teratogenic (malformations of fetuses).	Prescribed drug that can effect second and third generations of offspring.
Plasticizers (BPA)	Plastic softeners and antioxidants.	Plastic bottles, toys, cosmetics.

to endocrine disruptors as the cause of a declining alligator population in Lake Apopka, Florida. The alligators in this area have diminished reproductive organs that prevent successful reproduction. These problems were connected to a large pesticide spill several years earlier, and the alligators were found to have endocrine disrupting chemicals in their bodies and eggs.

These were the warnings Rachel Carson described nearly 50 years ago. The signs were present even then, yet advocates like Carson were dismissed. Fifty years later, animal research is showing some pretty serious health consequences because of exposure to endocrine disruptors. But this may be just a glimpse into what could be happening to human beings.

An example that validates the animal model of endocrine disruptors in humans is that of the drug DES (diethylstilbestrol). DES was introduced in 1947 as an FDA approved drug for miscarriages and banned in 1971. This drug is an estrogen mimic and, in the 1960's, was shown to actually cause birth defects in the infants of mothers who took the drug. DES has been banned but it remains a clear example of an endocrine disruptor and its impact on humans, specifically the developing baby.

Speculated human health effects of endocrine disruptors like DES include:

- Reproductive effects/birth defects
- Cancer
- Low sperm count/sexual dysfunction
- Heart disease
- Cognitive disorders
- Sex reversal
- Premature puberty
- Altered immune function

It is believed that the timing of exposure to DES and other endocrine disruptors is critical, especially in the case of developing fetuses and infants who may be the most vulnerable to the effects of environmental estrogens. However, which health effects are caused by what chemicals and in what doses at what time is still being debated. Bioaccumulation of chemicals within the body is also a legitimate concern.

Children are more vulnerable to endocrine disruptors, especially when it comes to the development of their organs and hormonal systems. This increased vulnerability has been a primary concern with phthalates and BPA exposure in children. In response to this concern, Canada and Europe banned BPA from baby bottles. Currently there is fear over toys containing phthalates since these chemicals can be absorbed through the skin and mouth, and eventually may their way into the blood stream.

EXPOSURE TO ENDOCRINE DISRUPTORS

Exposure to endocrine disruptors can occur through direct contact with pesticides and other chemicals or through ingestion of contaminated water, food, or air. Chemicals suspected of acting as endocrine disruptors are found in insecticides, herbicides and fungicides that are used in agriculture, golf courses, and in the home. Industrial workers can be exposed to chemicals such as detergents, resins, and plasticizers with endocrine disrupting properties.

Endocrine disruptors enter the air or water as a by-product of many chemical and manufacturing processes and when plastics and other materials are burned. Further, studies have found that endocrine disruptors can leach out of plastics, including the type of plastic used to make hospital intravenous bags. Many endocrine disruptors are persistent in the environment and accumulate in fat, so the greatest exposures come from eating fatty foods and fish from contaminated water.

THE NEUROTOXIC EFFECTS OF TOXINS

Just looking at the effects chemical toxins have on the endocrine system is enough to cause grave concern. Yet this is only one aspect of the dangers these pollutants cause; chemical toxins also affect the nervous system. There are dozens of studies showing that various environmental pollutants can negatively impact the nervous system, causing a broad spectrum of symptoms and medical problems.

The nervous system collects, processes, and acts upon information generated both within the body and from the outside environment. For example, the nervous system controls your breathing, which it can speed up or slow down depending on your activity (inside environment). It can also inform you if your surroundings are cold or hot (outside environment).

This incredible system that controls the body is divided into the central nervous system (CNS) which includes the spinal cord and brain, and peripheral nervous system (PNS) which includes all of the nerves outside the CNS. Nerve cells and neurotransmitters (chemicals that tell nerves what to do) make up the nervous system and are the sights where toxins can act directly or indirectly.

One of the reasons why toxins can easily affect our nervous system is because the majority of them are fat soluble, thus allowing them to easily penetrate our brains and nerves. This is one of the major problems with toxins; their ability to bioaccumulate over a period of time in fatty tissues. The nervous system is primarily made up of fatty tissue so the level of specific toxins can be high in this area of the body.

There are a number of ways toxins can damage the nervous system. They can disrupt the chemical balance, deteriorate nerve cells, and effect different cell structures that eventually negatively impact cell function.

As we discussed in Chapter 2, VOCs have been found in every person tested by the EPA. One of the problems with this fact is that VOCs have negative effects on both the PNS and the CNS. When they affect the CNS, this can lead to depression, mood disorders, irritability, and fatigue. Other symptoms may include memory loss, diminished cognitive function, reaction time, hand-eye coordination, and balance and gait disturbances. When VOCs affect the PNS, the symptoms may include tremors, numbness, and difficulty with fine motor movements.

Toxic metals can also have serious detrimental effects on the nervous system. Mercury is a neurotoxin capable of much damage. This toxin accumulates in the brain, entering cells, and impacting the way they function. Mercury in the brain is like getting viruses in your computer: Things just don't work properly after the infection. This heavy metal can also impact the levels of certain important brain chemicals (neurotransmitters) like serotonin and dopamine. Remember, serotonin is the feel-good chemical that is also important for proper sleep. Creating imbalances in brain chemicals like serotonin can have far reaching negative health effects.

SUPPORTING EVIDENCE

Since it would be unethical to give toxins to people just to study what happens, scientists often take another approach—looking at geographical areas where people have high exposure to environmental pollution. One such area is near Minamata City in Kumamoto Prefecture, Japan. This area is heavily polluted with methyl mercury (from a huge methyl mercury spill in the 1950's). In this analysis, 1,304 adults living in the polluted area were compared to 446 matched adults in a non-polluted area. The groups were surveyed for 64 subjective complaints. People in the polluted area reported a significantly higher prevalence for the following complaints: Stiffness, hand tremors, shrinking of upper arm musculature, arthralgia, insomnia, and lower back pain.

Even decades after the spill, the people living in the polluted area continue to exhibit a variety of symptoms not seen in the population that weren't subjected to the pollution. This has incredible far-reaching applications. How much of the pain we experience in our everyday lives can be linked to chemical toxins? The answer to this question is unknown but this comparison opens up many possibilities.

IMMUNE EFFECTS

The immune system is made up of specialized cells and organs that all work together to protect your body and keep you healthy. Specialized cells include the white blood cells which include macrophages that gobble up foreign invaders, T-cells that act as the warning bell for the immune system, B-cells which are the police (antibodies) that patrol the body, and a whole host of other important cells involved in a number of responses. The main organs of the immune system are the bone marrow (where blood cells are produced), the thymus gland (where T-cells mature) lymph nodes (detection and clean up centers), and the spleen (where antibody-coated bacteria are removed and red blood cells destroyed). When this system is optimal your body is well protected from most conditions including cancer.

But when the immune system is not functioning optimally, you are at risk for infections and other immune related conditions. Most of the time we blame it on stress or a lack of sleep. But how many times have we blamed it on environmental toxins? Perhaps we should. Environmental toxins can have a wide range of effects on the immune system. They can slow down the immune systems' reaction to bacteria and viruses, making you more susceptible to these infections. On the other hand, they can have a stimulating impact on T-cells, making them more sensitive to foreign material and eventually leading to allergies and autoimmune diseases.

Polycyclic aromatic hydrocarbons (PAHs) are chemicals created by combustion that can depress not only white blood cells but also some of the immune system organs. We are exposed to PAHs from the burning of fuels including oil and coal, as well as in various foods we consume.

Pesticides can also have a very detrimental impact on the immune system. Many autoimmune issues have been linked to chronic pesticide exposure, especially people working with and around these chemicals. Remember that pesticides are also found in up to 90 percent of all the foods consumed in the United States.

CANCER

We don't have to look far to conclude that environmental toxins are a contributing factor to the spread of cancer. In fact, the *British Medical Journal*, a respected scientific publication, noted that 75 percent of all cancers are environmentally induced. Six years earlier, the *Journal of the National Cancer Institute* stated that over 90 percent of all cancers are environmentally induced and that less than five percent had anything to do with genetics.

The evidence on endocrine disruptors alone gives us plenty of evidence that toxins in the environment contribute to cancer. Certain estrogen metabolites (the breakdown products of estrogen) such as 16-hydroxy- and 4-hydro- estrogens have been linked to cancer. The tremendous influx of endocrine disruptors that include estrogen mimickers like BPA create more estrogen in the body and this can lead to higher levels of these estrogen byproducts which can ultimately trigger hormone-dependant cancer.

Over the last ten years there has definitely been a push toward gaining a better understanding of what causes cancer. And environmental toxins have taken center stage in this campaign. There is now little doubt that environmental toxins are a contributing factor to cancer. Pesticides, heavy metals, PCBs, and a whole portfolio of compounds are at the core of what drives the growth of this disease.

THE NEXT STEP

There are a number of questions that often come up when discussing environmental medicine. One question is whether or not chemical toxins are accumulating in our bodies and what effect that pollution can have on us biophysically. We have without doubt shown that every human being is carrying a toxic burden. Even the doubters can't argue this point. But what they haven't accepted is the effects of these toxins on human health. To determine your exposure to toxins, visit my website www.drgaetano.com and take the "Are You Toxic?" quiz.

Hundreds of published papers support the fact that environmental toxins are indeed causing harm. Wildlife observations, human studies, and the fact that we aren't solving many of the health issues we are now confronted with point to the fact that chemicals toxins may be having a major effect on human physiology. The next step is to determine how we can become better equipped to detoxify these harmful chemicals.

5

Mechanisms of Detoxification

THE HUMAN BODY HAS FOUR MAIN excretory pathways that remove environmental toxins (exogenous toxins) as well as toxic products produced by the body (endogenous toxins). These include the feces, urine, sweat, and breath. Although some toxins get eliminated directly by these pathways, many toxins need to be transformed into water soluble compounds. Still others have to be changed into complex molecules. These transformations and changes occur in the most important detoxification organ in the body, the liver. Other organ systems involved in detoxification include the kidneys, gastrointestinal tract, and the skin.

THE WAYS TOXINS EXIT THE BODY

An often forgotten pathway of toxin excretion is the breath. If you have ever run into someone who has consumed a great deal of alcohol you can usually smell it on their breath. This is also the way you can measure someone's blood alcohol levels. Alcohol breath analyzer tests use the breath as a measure of blood alcohol levels.

Obviously, the lungs remove more than just alcohol. In fact, we can consider carbon dioxide a toxin that is eliminated from the body every time you exhale. The main job of the lungs is to take in oxygen and exchange it for carbon dioxide. Having healthy lungs is not only important for this function but also for the elimination of some toxic chemicals accumulating in our bodies.

Our bodies begin to sweat when we get hot in order to maintain normal body temperature. This can occur due to external temperature changes created by a sauna or during aerobic exercise. When body temperature is increased because of these or other factors, the body naturally begins to sweat. Sweat consists of a number of compounds that include water, lactate, urea, and a number of minerals such as sodium, potassium, calcium, magnesium, copper, and zinc. Some of the compounds in sweat are similar to those found in urine, making the skin much like the kidneys. When the body is heated, some toxic chemicals like xenobiotics and heavy metals can be excreted via this large organ. During times of elevated body temperature, toxic chemicals are loosened from fat tissues, some get released into the blood while others exit through the skin.

Urine is another well known excretion pathway. All humans view urination in this way but few think that it eliminates other toxic chemicals beside uric acid. To understand some of the chemicals that are eliminated in urine, all we have to do is recall the number of times we hear about steroid use among athletes. When they are tested for these compounds, it is always urinary testing that exposes the abusers.

In environmental medicine, testing for heavy metals like mercury, lead or cadmium requires analysis of not only the blood, but also the feces and/or the urine because these are both important excretory pathways. The kidneys not only excrete direct water soluble compounds, they also excrete chemicals that have been prepared by Phase II detoxification in the liver. Phase II converts fat soluble compounds into more water soluble versions that can enter the urine and be excreted out of the body. Healthy functioning kidneys are important in producing urine and eliminating toxins.

As we've just mentioned, the feces is an important route of excretion for chemical toxins. When toxins go through Phase I and II detoxification pathways in the liver they are carried into the gastrointestinal tract by bile. Once the bile gets into the intestinal tract via the duodenum, most of it will be re-absorbed unless soluble fiber is present. Soluble fiber binds the bile and both get excreted out of the body through the feces. However, in order for the body to properly eliminate these chemicals through the feces and the urine we need to have an optimally functioning liver.

THE LIVER (PHASE I AND PHASE II)

Located in the right upper quadrant of the abdominal cavity, the liver is the largest internal organ of the body (the largest overall organ is the skin). One of the interesting aspects of the liver is that it receives a dual blood supply: The portal vein brings blood from the gastrointestinal tract and spleen while the hepatic artery brings fresh oxygenated blood from the heart. The hepatic vein then brings metabolized and detoxified blood back to the heart for redistribution throughout the body.

The human liver carries out over 500 different metabolic functions including the detoxification of harmful substances from the body. Over two quarts of blood pass through this important organ every minute of every day, filtering and transforming chemicals to keep the body clean. The liver also produces bile into which fat-soluble toxins are attached and then discharged into the gastrointestinal tract.

Bile has two major functions in body. The first is for the emulsification of fats and the second is to carry toxins and other wastes from the liver into the duodenum (first section of the small intestine). Since fats aren't water soluble, bile emulsifies them so they are capable of getting into the blood stream for transport.

Bile also contains a majority of the body's metabolic wastes including dead blood cells and toxic chemicals like pesticides. Once formed, bile, along with its waste products and processed toxins, moves from the liver to the gallbladder. It is then secreted into the intestine where it is used for the absorption of fats and to help with stool movement. It is also here that bile and its toxic load are picked up by dietary fiber and excreted out of the body through the feces. A lack of dietary fiber will result in inadequate binding, allowing toxins to be re-absorbed. Therefore, one of the most important ways of improving detoxification is to have plenty of dietary fiber in the diet.

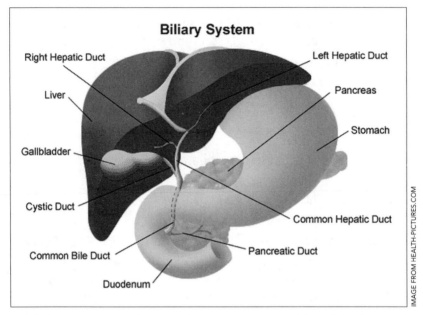

FIGURE 5.1 Anatomy of liver and relationship with gall bladder and duodenum

PACKAGING TOXINS FOR EXPORT

The liver's primary goal when confronted with a toxic chemical is to neutralize it (making it water soluble). Most toxins are fat soluble, which means they are difficult to get rid of, just like an ink stain on your shirt. If elevated levels of toxins are present because of poor detoxification, a majority of them can end up being stored in adipose tissue (fat) and cell membranes throughout the body (cell membranes are made up of fats). Sometimes they can stay dormant in tissues for decades, but other times—because of various activities—they can be released. For example, during periods of weight loss, exercise, stress, and fasting, these chemicals are released into the blood stream, possibly leading to negative reactions throughout the body.

A recent controlled study demonstrated that when a group of overweight people went on a diet, their reduction in body fat correlated with an increase in circulating pesticides (pesticides are stored in fat tissue). The end result was that the pesticides reduced circulating active thyroid hormone (T3) thus giving rise to a reduced metabolic rate. Could this be the reason why people on weight loss programs plateau?

A complex network of detoxification mechanisms inside liver cells are capable of processing drugs, hormones, steroids, chemicals, pesticides, and almost every possible toxin imaginable. Phase I enzymes transform these toxins into water-soluble molecules so they can be easily be excreted by the kidney and reactive forms for Phase II enzymes where these chemicals are conjugated. The reactive forms are actually free radicals which are, at times, more dangerous than the original toxin. Therefore, it is critically important to make sure these Phases, especially Phase II, function optimally.

SIMPLIFYING PHASE I AND II

Phase I and II detoxification pathways have seldom been easy to understand. Many detoxification books don't spend a lot of time on them because of this very issue. Even during my early medical school years, there was always some confusion about the body's detoxification pathways. Yet these pathways are very important to understand because being able to support them is a valuable part of purifying the body from chemical toxins. As we have already learned, the only way to reduce our body burden is not only to reduce exposure but also to improve our body's ability to get rid of toxins. The best way to accomplish this is with a thorough understanding of Phase I and II pathways.

Sometimes you have to wonder why we have these pathways, but a general understanding of the properties of toxins puts this into perspective. The majority of toxins are fat soluble, which makes them very difficult to eliminate. Its like trying to get an oil stain off your shirt with water—it just can't be done unless you use detergent. Phase I and II change these toxins allowing them to be removed from the body.

An analogy that seems to work with my audiences is the oil paint, turpentine, and cloth comparison. If you are painting a fence with an oil-based paint, you'll probably get some of the paint on your hands. Once that paint has dried on your skin you can't get it off with water. What you need to do is dissolve that paint with turpentine. Doing this

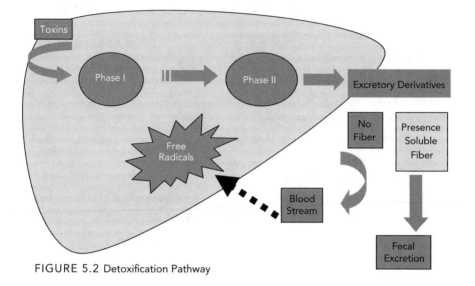

FIGURE 5.2 Detoxification Pathway

creates a mixture of paint and turpentine that can be easily wiped off with a cloth. You then throw the paint-stained cloth in the trash to wait until it can be transported to the dump.

This is very similar to what happens in Phase I and II detoxification pathways. Phase I is the turpentine dissolving the paint and creating a new solution on your hand. Phase II is the cloth that binds the solution and eliminates it from the hands for excretion.

PHASE I PATHWAY

This first part of the liver's detoxification pathway involves biotransformation. Much like the turpentine dissolving the paint and transforming it to a new solution, Phase I accomplishes the same kind of thing.

The Phase I detoxification pathway involves more than 100 enzymes known as the cytochrome P450. These enzymes each have

---

Enzymes are mainly proteins, generated by your body that control the speed of biochemical reactions. They are known as a biological catalyst or initiators of reactions. Without enzymes, all reactions in the body would come to a standstill.

---

specificity for one or more of the chemical toxins they come in contact with. They change these toxins in such a way that Phase II can then neutralize them and give them an easy exit out of the body.

An important thing to keep in mind is that there is genetic variability within the P450 family of enzymes from one person to the next. This means that the rate at which some of these enzymes work may vary from one person to the next. This creates different constitutions in people, which will make some sensitive and others resistant to various toxins. Examples are people who can't handle alcohol and become intoxicated even with the smallest amount. Some people can't tolerate caffeine—it makes them jittery and keeps them awake. Others, however, have absolutely no problem with caffeine. The difference in these individuals is all in the P450 system diversity.

This pathway is like a double edged sword because it converts toxic chemicals into less harmful chemicals—yet, if overactive, it can produce extremely toxic free radicals. Antioxidants like glutathione can actually disengage free radicals, making them harmless. However, if these antioxidants are lacking and exposure is high, these toxic chemicals become even more dangerous then they were at the start of the process. When this happens, reactions begin occurring in different parts of the liver and body. In fact some of these substances can do so much harm that they can cause cancer.

Another thing that can happen in Phase I is that, if an excessive amount of toxins are ingested, the cytochrome p450 system can be stimulated and become overactive. This is known as induction of Phase I and will lead to high levels of damaging free radicals. Substances that can cause this to happen include caffeine, alcohol, dioxins, saturated fats, pesticides, barbiturates, paint fumes, sulfonamides, and exhaust fumes. If Phase II can't keep up with this bombardment, serious consequences can result.

PHASE II PATHWAY

Phase II is known as the conjugation pathway and, as its name suggests, it basically adds another substance to the toxic chemical or drug to make it less harmful. This makes the toxin water soluble so it can easily be excreted out of the body, either through the urine or bile. Through conjugation reactions, the liver is able to turn hormones, drugs, and toxins into substances that can be eliminated from the body. Phase II acts like the bomb squad that arrives to disengage the bombs.

There are six main forms of Phase II detoxification paths that include acetylation, amino acid conjugation, glucuronidation, methylation, glutathione conjugation, and sulfation. Each one of these forms removes specific types of toxins and requires specific nutrients for their optimal functionality. Think of each of these paths as specialized bomb squads, each trained to disengage specific types of bombs.

ACETYLATION: A compound known as Acetyl-coenzyme A is the main element in acetylation reactions. This Phase II reaction binds and eliminates sulfa drugs, which includes the vast array of sulfur-based antibiotics. In order for this reaction to occur, vitamin C, pantothenic acid, and thiamine are essential. These nutrients are also involved in energy production.

AMINO ACID CONJUGATION: As the name suggests, this type of conjugation reaction involves the attachment of amino acids to the toxin. The main amino acids that bind and neutralize the toxins are arginine, glutamine, glycine, ornithine, and taurine. Most of these amino acids can be obtained from protein. For this reason, a diet that contains a good supply of protein is important to detoxification.

GLUCURONIDATION: This conjugation reaction involves attaching glucuronic acid to a toxin. Most prescription drugs and food additives are detoxified this way. Limonene, the active ingredient in citrus rind, can enhance glucuronidation.

GLUTATHIONE CONJUGATION: Glutathione is the body's most powerful antioxidant. It stops free radicals from doing harm in various areas of the human body, especially in the liver. Glutathione is made up of three amino acids: Glutamine, cysteine, and glycine. It is synthesize in the body although some dietary sources do exist.

Heavy metals and fat soluble toxins are the main binding substrates for glutathione. It is important to supply the body with antioxidant and nutritional products that can help keep the levels of glutathione healthy especially in the liver. If Phase I is overactive, this will cause a release of free radicals into the cell which will lead to glutathione being depleted.

METHYLATION: An important way of neutralizing toxins and inactivating damaging estrogen is a process called methylation. As the name suggests, methylation involves adding a methyl group to the toxin. A methyl group is simply a molecule made up of a one carbon atom and three hydrogen atoms. The process called methylation can neutralize toxins, especially estrogen metabolites. Estrogen metabolites are active forms of estrogens, some of which are carcinogenic. Methylation neutralizes these compounds, allowing them to be safely excreted out of the body. Nutritionals that can help this process included DIM (diindolylmethane), a substance derived from broccoli and Brussels sprouts, which is capable of neutralizing bad estrogen and creating healthy estrogen metabolites. S-adenosylmethionine (SAMe) can also be helpful in donating a methyl group and thus neutralizing toxins.

SULFATION: Sulfation is a process involving the addition of a sulfur group to a toxin, thereby neutralizing it. Neurotransmitters (communicating chemicals in the nervous system), steroid hormones, thyroid hormones, food additives, certain drugs, and intestinal bacterial toxins are neutralized by sulfation. You can enhance this conjugation reaction by eating a diet high in sulfur-containing foods like onions, garlic, broccoli, and Brussels sprouts.

Phase II can also be activated by certain compounds and slowed down by others. This becomes important when discussing scientific detoxification in the next chapter.

THE INTESTINES

The gastrointestinal tract plays a big role in detoxification, mainly because it receives toxins bound to bile acids for excretion. What happens to this bile will be directly related to what's in the intestinal tract. As we mentioned earlier, bile needs to be bound to dietary fiber for its quick exit out of the body through the feces.

If high enough levels of dietary fiber are not present, most of this bile will be reabsorbed back into the blood stream—along with the toxins it's trying to dump. This is why fasting may not be beneficial during detoxification. Fasting usually involves abstinence from food for two to sometimes 14 days. This can be problematic because fasting releases toxins stored in fatty tissue. These toxins will eventually make their way into the intestinal tract via bile acids. Unfortunately, without fiber, the bus to take them out of the body won't be there. Fasting usually means no fiber in the intestine, and no fiber means that the toxins will get reabsorbed back into the blood stream. Once they are back in the blood stream, they will either become incorporated into fatty tissues once again or cause direct damage to the tissues themselves.

THE KIDNEYS

The kidneys are another important organ in detoxification. They eliminate a number of toxic substances via Phase II reactions including caffeine, drugs, steroids and toxic metals. This is the reason why we test for toxic metals by taking urine samples. Toxic metals like mercury, lead, cadmium, and many others are eliminated by the kidneys through the urine.

Probably the best way to ensure optimal kidney function is something we call dilution. This means drinking plenty of purified water, which is the easiest and best way to keep the kidneys functioning optimally. Our recommendation is at least eight glasses of purified water daily as a starting point. Make sure you keep track of how much water you drink until it becomes habit.

THE SKIN

The skin is the largest organ in the body and has some detoxification properties. In the past, we assumed that a sauna only released toxins through sweat. But research has shown us that saunas mobilize toxins from fat cells. But, these toxins don't become part of the body's perspiration. Instead, they are released into the blood stream. Our recommendation is that if you embark on sauna treatments, make sure you are on the scientific detoxification program laid out in the next chapter so that these toxins will not be re-absorbed by the body.

Another way of mobilizing toxins is through exercise. Exercise not only mobilizes toxins through sweat, it also promotes the mobilization of toxins from adipose tissue. Again, this type of toxin mobilization needs be a part of the scientific detoxification program.

SUMMARY

Optimally functioning detoxification pathways are key components to overall well-being. The most important and complex aspects of these pathways are Phase I and II systems located in the liver. If Phase I and II detoxification pathways become overloaded, there will be a buildup of toxins in the body. The fat solubility of these toxins allows them to become incorporated into cell membranes and fatty tissues throughout the body where they can remain for years.

Common areas of accumulation include the endocrine glands (hormonal) and the brain, which may result in hormonal imbalances, brain dysfunction, PMS, early menopause, and autoimmune disease just to name a few. The key to avoiding these serious consequences is to minimize toxic exposure and insure optimal functionality of these pathways.

6

CHAPTER SIX

Digestion:
The Foundation of Healing

A SYSTEM VITAL TO THE PROCESS of detoxification is the gastrointestinal (GI) tract. It is in the GI tract where many toxins can be absorbed
and, at the same time, eliminated by the body. Unfortunately, when we
think of the GI tract, we often think of the stomach that fills up when
we eat and the elimination processes that doesn't always work as well
as we would like. We very seldom consider the intricacy of this part of
the body and its relationship to general health. Yet science is beginning
to uncover much about this critical system.

The GI tract does a lot more then just digest food, absorb nutrients, and eliminate waste. It plays a vital role in immune function, in
regulating sugar metabolism, in controlling cholesterol levels, and yes, in
detoxification. It is through the GI tract that toxins attached to foods and
liquids are absorbed into the body. Statistics tell us that, over a lifetime,
the average American will consume approximately 20 to 30 tons of food.
Food labels tell us that much of this food contains artificial fats, coloring agents, flavor additives, and preservatives. Much of the meat and
dairy we eat is tainted with hormones and antibiotics. A large amount
of the food we consume also harbors potentially harmful pesticide residue. How much of this is absorbed into your blood stream through
your GI tract?

When these food toxins are processed through the liver, a majority of them are excreted through the GI tract. In other words, the GI tract is really a gateway for the entrance and exit of chemical toxins. From this rather rudimentary knowledge, we can easily make the assumption that a healthy GI tract is critical for proper detoxification.

THE GUT-BRAIN CONNECTION

The GI tract has a close relationship with the brain—much closer than any of us would have imagined. Research shows that the brain and gut share many of the same hormones and neurotransmitters. This may partly explain why stress and emotions often trigger gastrointestinal problems.

Think about certain situations that make you nauseous, ongoing stress that causes ulcers, and emotional moments that give us butterflies. All of these reactions begin in the brain and have symptoms that express themselves in the gut. Many aspects of stress and other emotional problems can give rise to all sorts of GI complaints. That's because the brain and the gastrointestinal system are intimately connected.

The latest research shows that the entire journey that food takes through the 30-foot long GI tract is controlled by a remarkable communication network known as the enteric nervous system (ENS). This intricate nerve complex is located in the gut wall and communicates with the brain via the spinal cord. In turn, hormones, neurotransmitters, and connections to the central nervous system affect muscles, mucosa, and blood vessels in the digestive tract which then influences the ENS. In his book, *The Second Brain*, Michael Gershon, M.D., calls the gut the second brain. He claims that over 100 million neurotransmitters line the length of the gut from the esophagus to the colon; that's equal to the number found in the brain. Nearly every hormone and neurotransmitter found in the brain is also found in the gut.

HEALING BEGINS IN THE GUT

It has been said that the digestive tract is the caveat of all healing. This is a statement I repeat often in my lectures because it is so true. Healing must first occur in this vital part of the body before any other place.

If clinical practice has taught me one thing, it is the fact that the GI tract is the shelter that protects us from the elements and ultimately plays a big role in whether or not we maintain a level of well being. How is this possible? In this chapter, we will begin an investigation of how the GI tract works and what can happen when it is compromised. You will, in the end, have a different appreciation of this amazing tunnel, and ultimately, because of what you learn, you will have a much improved chance of properly detoxifying your body.

We can clearly state that you CAN NOT detoxify until the digestive tract is in order. Digestive function must be working optimally for detoxification to work. Without proper GI function, the body will have a difficult time eliminating toxic waste. Not only will this create more toxicities, it may cause serious side effects.

A TRIP THROUGH THE TUBE (ANATOMY AND PHYSIOLOGY)

The digestive tract is made up of a long tube with specific parts all participating in the process of digestion and elimination. It begins in the mouth, followed by the esophagus, which opens into the stomach. The stomach is followed by the duodenum—the 12 finger length part of the small intestine that includes the jejunum and ileum. The last section is the large intestine, including both rectum and colon.

Role of the Mouth and Esophagus

The first part of the digestive tract is the mouth. This is where food is crushed and chewed. Food is mixed with saliva to create a smooth bolus that can move down the esophagus into the stomach. During this process, some digestion does occur since saliva contains some amylases that break down carbohydrates.

Role of the Stomach

The stomach is an important part of digestion, since it is here that the food is churned, and where hydrochloric acid and the enzyme pepsin are secreted to begin the process of digestion. These factors are important for proper protein digestion and mineral absorption. Generally speaking, the process takes anywhere from 45 minutes to four hours to complete and make its way into the small intestine.

A couple of things to remember is that during digestion, the pH of the stomach drops to an incredible level of 1.2 (pH ranges from 1-14, with 1 being the most acid). This is an extremely acidic level, so strong that it could dissolve a nail and easily burn through human tissues. Yet this potent acid doesn't burn holes in the stomach wall.

When we look at the histology of the stomach, we find it contains many mucous cells. These cells produce a substance called mucin that actually coats the stomach and neutralizes the acid as it tries to come in contact with the stomach wall. It is the mucin that protects the stomach wall and prevents this acid from burning holes in our digestive tract.

Being a curious mind, I wanted to know why the stomach pH had to be so acidic. The answers were simple, but very important to understand since many stomach disorders are treated by changing this pH. For example, antacids increase the pH, significantly making the stomach less acidic.

Mother Nature creates this high acid environment for a number of reasons. The two most important are to begin breaking down proteins and to kill potential toxins before the food moves into the lower bowel. Stomach pH is low enough to kill most micro-organisms including Candida, yeast, and even parasites

By altering this pH with antacids or prescriptions like H2-antag-onists and proton pump inhibitors, you will ultimately change the gut environment. This is dangerous because it will allow unfriendly micro-organisms to enter the body and inhibit protein digestion.

Role of the Small Intestine

It takes food approximately two to four hours to make its way through the small intestine. The small intestine is made up of three different parts: The duodenum, the jejunum, and the ileum. Together, these three parts are nearly 21 feet long. The duodenum is the first part of the small intestine and is almost 12 inches in length, followed by the jeju-num (8 feet) and finally the ileum (12 feet).

THE DUODENUM: An important part of the small intestine, the duodenum is where much secretion, absorption, and digestion occur. As soon as the chyme (a mass of partially-digested food) moves into the duodenum, signals are sent to the pancreas to release pancreatic enzymes. Each day the pancreas secretes nearly 1.5 quarts of pancreatic juice into the small intestine. These enzymes include proteases, lipases, amylases, and other compounds that help break down foods. Without the release of these enzymes, digestion and absorption could not occur.

The enzymes released by the pancreas include lipases which, along with bile, help in the digestion of fats. Lipase deficiencies and bile secretion problems can result in the malabsorption of fats and fat soluble vitamins. Amylases function to break carbohydrates down into simple sugars for absorption. Weight loss products like starch blockers work by inhibiting the effectiveness of this enzyme. The proteases—including trypsin, chymotrypsin, and carboxypeptidase—are also secreted by the pancreas and break proteins down into amino acids. When proteins are not completely digested, bacteria in the lower bowel act on these particles, creating toxic compounds that can wreak havoc on gastrointestinal health. Proteases also work to keep the small intestine free from parasites, Candida, and all sorts of other invasive organisms.

BILE: Another event that occurs in the duodenum is the release of bile from both the gall bladder and the liver. This is important because it allows fat soluble food particles to be absorbed into the blood stream. Bile acts as an emulsifier, allowing this important process to occur. Think of bile much like soap. When you get an oil stain on a shirt, you can't simply remove it with water; you need to use soap. Soap allows water soluble compounds to mix with fat soluble ones. Bile does the same thing with food substances.

Another important function of the duodenum is the absorption of minerals. Minerals predominantly get absorbed here in an acidic environment. When people are on over-the-counter or prescription drugs like antacids, H2-antagonists (Zantac) or proton pump inhibitors (Nexium), problems arise. Because these products create an alkaline environment, mineral absorption is inhibited, causing deficiencies.

This could prevent calcium, magnesium, zinc, and all sorts of other important minerals from being absorbed.

JEJUNUM & ILEUM: The jejunum is the part of the small intestine where water soluble vitamins, carbohydrates, and proteins are absorbed. Following this eight foot long tube is the ileum, where fat soluble vitamins and fats are absorbed. One interesting aspect of the ileum is that, in its distal end, vitamin B-12 is also absorbed through intrinsic factor.

Role of Large Intestine

The large intestine, often referred to as the colon, measures about five feet in length. Water and electrolytes (various salts) are absorbed into the blood stream while waste products from digestion are temporarily stored in the colon before elimination takes place.

One big problem in the colon is the slow removal of waste products. The term "constipation" describes this problem—one that is suffered by a large percentage of the population. Patients that come to my clinic often tell me they have regular bowel movements. The problem is that they think that a bowel movement every three to four days is normal. This is where we need re-education. Bowel movements should occur daily. In fact, one should have a couple of bowel movements every day for healthy GI function.

Stagnation can cause the build up of toxic materials, causing damage to the wall of the colon. This, in turn, can lead to a number of GI problems including hemorrhoids, diverticulitis, irritable bowel syndrome, and even colon cancer. The way to keep the colon healthy is by ensuring ample amounts of fruits and vegetables that provide lots of dietary fiber. Fiber is a vital nutrient that can keep you regular and provide a whole slew of health benefits.

DETERIORATION OF GI HEALTH

When we look at the diet of the average American, we see foods high in saturated fat and refined carbohydrates, low in fresh fruits and vegetables, and large in portion sizes. The end result is an unhealthy way of eating that can lead to digestive problems.

FIGURE 6.1

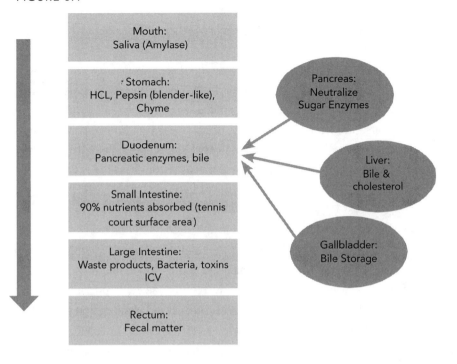

The Western diet refers to the dietary habits of people living in the industrialized countries of the world. Westernization refers to the gradual change that took us from an diet filled with unrefined plant foods to one rich in meat, dairy, sugar, and processed foods. This type of diet is now linked to the development of many of the chronic diseases of the 21st century.

The origins of the changes can be traced back to the beginning of the industrial revolution, when most people lived in rural areas and cities weren't the metropolises they have now become. In those days, most food substances were purchased either through a local farmer who lived within walking distance or grown in one's own backyard. Grocery stores were only used for particular staples like flour and spices. Again, this was a small collection of items, since preservation of food through artificial agents hadn't really been introduced on a large scale. Overall, most foods consumed were natural and contained most of their nutrients. Flavoring agents, fats and sugars were not consumed in large amounts. As a result, people ate diets where dietary fiber loads were higher, fat and sugar content much lower.

Contrast that with today's average diet. Our grocery stores carry over 30,000 food items, most of which are tainted with preservative, saturated fats, and sugar to improve flavor. The average North American consumes nearly 150 pounds of sugar per year and over 50 pounds of high fructose corn syrup, often through soft drinks. Our diet has drastically changed—and so has the health of our bodies.

DIETARY EFFECTS ON THE HUMAN BODY

Our Western diet, which is a drastic deviation from the diet of our ancestors, has had monumental effects on the human body. Remember we are made from the nutrients we consume. They, in turn, make up the structure of every single cell in the body. How those cells function and feel will reflect how we function and feel. How those cells function and feel is predicated on the quality and type of nutrients they are given.

The Western diet is rich in saturated fats, sugars, and chemicals that do little to support cellular function. This has negative effects on the cell's membranes, its organelles, and its DNA. As a result, alterations to a number of crucial nutritional characteristics can occur within the human body. These altered nutritional characteristics include glycemic load, macronutrient composition, fatty acid composition, micronutrient density, and fiber content. Each one of these has dramatically changed since humans first inhabited the earth, and those changes are at the heart of many degenerative diseases.

The glycemic index came onto the nutritional scene in the 1980's. It was—and continues to be—used as a relative comparison of the blood sugar-raising potential of various foods. The measure we call glycemic load is one of the nutritional characteristics that has changed greatly since our ancestral roots. Consider this fact alone, that our Western culture has gone from consuming negligible refined sugars to nearly 150 pounds of sugar per year. The end result has been tremendous stress on our sugar regulating apparatus, which has led to the dramatic rise in diabetes.

TABLE 6.1 Nutritional Characteristic Changes And Their Possible Effects

Nutritional Characteristic	Substances Involved	Effects
Glycemic load	Refined sugars, carbohydrates	Diabetes, hypoglycemia
Macronutrient composition	Proteins, fats, carbohydrates	Cardiovascular disease, obesity
Fatty acid composition	Saturated fats, trans fats	Cardiovascular disease, cancer
Micronutrient density	Vitamins, minerals	Cardiovascular disease, immune dysfunction, chronic degenerative diseases
Fiber content	Dietary fiber (soluble and insoluble)	Cardiovascular disease, diabetes, obesity, cancer, immune dysfunction

Our macronutrient composition intake has also changed, going from a high protein, complex carbohydrate diet to one high in saturated fats and simple sugars. The quality of these macronutrients has also changed putting even more stress on the cells they are suppose to support.

One area that has received a lot of attention recently is fatty acid composition, particularly in light of the vast amount of research that's been done on omega-3 fatty acids. The Western diet usually contains excessive amounts of saturated and trans fatty acids and very little omega-3 fatty acids. If we look at this historically we again find a dramatic shift from our ancestors, whose high plant diet contained large amounts of omega-3 fatty acids and negligible amounts of saturated and trans fats. This shift in fatty acid consumption has contributed to the development of obesity and cardiovascular disease including elevations in cholesterol levels.

One category that is well accepted by the majority of Americans is micronutrient density. This refers to the vitamin and mineral content of foods. It is no secret that the micronutrient content of most foods has dramatically dropped in the last 200 years. The introduction of new agricultural practices, including use of fertilizers and pesticides, has lowered the nutrient content of most foods. This has led to the popularity of multi-vitamin mineral supplements.

Probably the most important nutritional shift receiving the least amount of attention is dietary fiber. Fiber content in the American diet has dropped considerably. The USDA estimates that the average American consumes about 15 grams of fiber per day; a considerable difference from the daily 25-30 gram requirement. But is the daily requirement even accurate if we compare it to ancestral diets? The answer is probably no.

Fiber consumption should be higher in Western cultures since it has so many beneficial effects on human health. We are talking about a nutrient that not only can reduce the risk of cardiovascular disease and diabetes, it can actually help people lose weight and even reduce cancer.

The alteration in nutritional characteristics is really at the heart of many of the chronic diseases that plague Western civilization. But there is even more that many of us haven't considered. One problem that hasn't been addressed is that all of this food places an enormous burden on the digestive tract. The GI tract was originally made to consume foods rich in nutrients and enzymes that are also relatively easy to digest. In the last 100 years we've introduced foods that are difficult to digest, foods lacking their own enzymes, and foods that cause inhibitory effects on our body's own enzyme systems. The end result is that we have created the beginnings of digestive fall out.

DIGESTIVE FALL OUT

Figure 3 paints a complete picture of what happens when digestive fall out occurs. If you follow the diagram, you'll see that the end result is chronic disease. The first part of declining digestive health is caused by a lack of digestive enzyme due to a number of contributing factors. Poor diet, high levels of free radicals, and stress can all cause a reduction in enzyme production.

For example, when one is under stress (fight or flight response), one of the systems that slows down is the sympathetic nervous system response in the digestive tract. When you are stressed, your digestion will not function properly because the nervous system is tells the body to slow down the blood supply to that area. The end result is a reduction in circulation and thus a reduction in the overall activity of the GI tract.

FIGURE 6.2 Declining Digestive Health

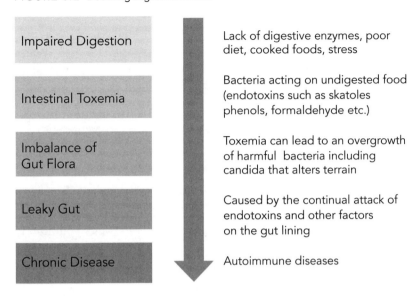

Impaired Digestion	Lack of digestive enzymes, poor diet, cooked foods, stress
Intestinal Toxemia	Bacteria acting on undigested food (endotoxins such as skatoles phenols, formaldehyde etc.)
Imbalance of Gut Flora	Toxemia can lead to an overgrowth of harmful bacteria including candida that alters terrain
Leaky Gut	Caused by the continual attack of endotoxins and other factors on the gut lining
Chronic Disease	Autoimmune diseases

This will also reduce the amount of enzymes secreted, which will cause undigested food particles to move down the digestive tract. Bacteria will act on these particles, creating endotoxins (toxins produced by organisms in the GI tract) that may include formaldehyde, skatoles, and indoles. These chemicals will create problems in the GI tract that will result in an imbalance in the friendly bacteria lining the digestive tract walls. This reduction in friendly bacteria will allow the growth of bad bacteria and other harmful organisms like Candida. The end result is not a good one, as these events cause damage to the intestinal wall giving rise to something we call "leaky gut." Leaky gut occurs when the lining of the small intestine becomes permeable. This permeability allows large particles to get into the blood stream, causing immune reactions which can eventually lead to autoimmune disease.

LEAKY GUT

When the gut lining becomes altered or damaged, causing an increase in gastrointestinal permeability, the condition is called leaky gut syndrome. This injury can be caused by a number of contributing factors including antibiotics, yeast, Candida, bacteria, poor diet, and parasites. The damage can then cause the permeation of toxins, microbes, undigested food particles, waste, and other larger than normal macromolecules to enter the blood stream. This whole process has been linked to a number of growing health conditions, many of which are linked to the body's immune response to the absorbed compound.

Probably one of the most overlooked areas in gastrointestinal health is its importance in keeping harmful compounds from entering the blood stream. Most people are rather surprised when they learn about the structure of this barrier. It's surprising because what separates what's in your gut from getting into your blood is a wall that is just one cell layer thick! Think about that—a microscopic unit is all that keeps the gunk in your intestines from entering your blood. It's a testament to the incredible machine that is the human body.

When you have an accumulation of toxic waste in your intestine that hangs around for long periods because of a lack of fiber, these substances start damaging this one cell barrier. They start breaking it down and, in the end, cause perforations, or holes, in the gut wall. This allows a broad range of substances to leak into the blood stream. These substances—because they are foreign—are not recognized by the blood, so the immune system launches an attack. This reaction usually involves the formation of antibodies which can become confused and attack specific parts of the body. For example, some of these antibodies are sometimes mistaken for joint cartilage. One disease that evolves from this situation is rheumatoid arthritis an autoimmune condition that targets the joints. In another case, the antibodies can affect the skin, causing eczema.

Now just for a moment, let's imagine having leaky gut syndrome and trying to detoxify at the same time. As you move toxins from various stored areas into the liver for excretion through the GI tract, you can see how problems could arise. Increased gut permeability will allow some of these toxins to enter the blood stream, causing even more damage than when they were dormant in fatty tissue.

TESTING FOR LEAKY GUT

Diagnosing a leaky gut is not difficult. It simply requires using two types of sugars—mannitol and lactulose. Neither of these sugars are metabolized, meaning they are not broken down, so they can be easily measured in the urine.

Mannitol is a small sugar molecule easily absorbed by intestinal cells while lactulose is a large sugar molecule not easily absorbed. However, if someone has leaky gut syndrome, the space between intestinal cells will be larger, allowing lactulose to be more easily absorbed. By utilizing both of these sugars, mannitol serves as a marker for general absorption while lactulose serves as an indicator of increased intestinal permeability.

The testing involves taking both sugars orally and testing the urine six hours later. In a normal situation, the mannitol recovered should be between five and 25 percent. The percentage of lactulose should be between 0.1 and 0.8 percent. If the levels of these sugars are higher, that indicates increased intestinal permeability. On the other hand, if they are lower, it could indicate a case of malabsorption.

THE GI ENVIRONMENT

When we talk about the gastrointestinal environment we are referring to the biological terrain of the gut. The biological terrain of the GI tract is similar to the soil a farmer plants his seeds in. That soil needs to have the right pH levels. The minerals need to be in balance and there needs to be a healthy number of bacteria in the soil. If all of these criteria are met then the farmer is in a much improved position to yield a healthy crop.

The gastrointestinal tract is similar in that it also needs to have a healthy terrain. Hydrochloric acid needs to be present in the stomach as do pancreatic enzymes in the duodenum. This is essential so that incomplete protein digestion doesn't occur, which can lead to intestinal toxemia.

The gut also needs to have the right amount of friendly bacteria. Probiotics are essential for GI health and optimal levels are a must for

a healthy gut environment. These bacteria have many functions including maintaining proper pH levels, preventing the overgrowth of bad
bacteria, creating beneficial gut products like short-chain fatty acids,
and helping support overall immune function.

Altering the gut environment at any time can lead to all sorts of
medical conditions, some of which can be very serious. Healthy gut
flora are so beneficial that recent scientific research shows that supplementing with probiotics may boost gum health, improve digestion,
enhance the immune system, and possibly protect against cancer.

THE IMMUNE SYSTEM

The immune system is a complex array of cells that help protect the
body from foreign invaders. It is made up of many different types of
immune cells with specific functions. As stated earlier, macrophages
act as scavengers by eating up bacteria and viruses that enter the
blood stream. T-cells are a kind of alarm system cell that communicates with B-cells, which are antibody forming cells. One way of
looking at this is that if a burglar comes in the house, the alarm system goes off (T-cell). This sends a signal to the police station (B-cell),
which send out the calvary of police officers (antibodies) to capture
the burglar.

An interesting aspect of the immune system that we don't give
much thought to is that between 70 and 80 percent of it is located in
the gut. This isn't something we think much about yet it adds another
enormous responsibility on this already very intricate system. So why
does Mother Nature put such a large part of the immune system in this
already busy area? To answer this question, let's go back to the burglar
breaking into the house. If you were given a couple of security person-
nel to guard your house from the burglar, where would you put them?
Probably at the front and back doors. In the same way, the immune system locates itself in the entry points where viruses, bacteria, toxins and
other invading organisms and substances could enter to cause damage
to the body. Since the GI tract is the biggest entry point of the body, the
immune keeps itself there.

HOW THE GI SYSTEM HELPS GET RID OF TOXINS

We've discussed the GI tract in depth because it plays a very important role in detoxification. For one, it can act as a barrier against toxins from entering the blood stream. This is why it's important to maintain a healthy blood-gut barrier; impaired digestion can break down this barrier, allowing the entry of foreign compounds.

Secondly, it is the gut that receives the neutralized toxins bound in bile for excretion. Generally speaking, the gut can not only act as the gateway for toxins entering the body but also for them leaving.

BILE, THE CARRIER

As I've mentioned in earlier chapters, bile collects neutralized toxins and carries them out of the liver into the gallbladder for storage. During a meal, when food enters the duodenum, one of the reactions triggered is the release of bile from both the gallbladder and liver. The bile enters the duodenum and mixes with the bolus of food. The whole mess then begins its journey down the intestinal tube.

As the bile moves down the GI tract, 98 percent of it will be reabsorbed into the blood stream. If you think about that for a moment, you'll see how confusing it is. If bile, with all the toxins attached, gets re-circulated back into the body, haven't we just defeated the goal of eliminating toxins? Of course we have. This scenario offers a clue to the important role fiber plays. Bile will not get reabsorbed if soluble fiber is present in the GI tract. Soluble fiber—found in oatmeal, barley, beans, nuts, and flaxseed—binds bile and holds it until the body eliminates it.

CREATING A HEALTHY GUT: THE A'S, B'S AND C'S

Creating a healthy gut that can both digest food and efficiently get rid of toxins is achievable. The digestive tract is one of the most responsive systems in the body and nutritional support can often result in very quick results. One reason may be because the digestive tract is constantly turning over.

Changing the diet is at the foundation of digestive renewal. You must reduce the consumption of unhealthy fats (trans fats and saturated fats), reduce refined carbohydrates, and increase the consumption of fresh fruits and vegetables. It's also wise to reduce coffee and alcohol consumption.

Supplements are also important, especially digestive enzymes, DGL, and probiotics. Taken over a short period of time, these products can help turn around your digestion by creating a healthy, functioning gut.

DIGESTIVE ENZYMES: Digestive enzymes are produced by the pancreas and secreted into the duodenum when you eat. They help the body break down food so the nutrients are separated and digested into absorbable molecules. Enzymes include proteases that break down proteins, lipases that break down fats, and amylases that break down carbohydrates. Without these enzymes, we could not break down the foods we eat, nutrient absorption would be impossible, and the end result would be a malnourished body, no matter how much food you consumed.

As we discussed earlier, a number of factors can contribute to a deficiency in enzyme production. Things like stress, poor diet, lack of exercise, and the use of prescription drugs can have a detrimental effect on enzyme production. This ultimately results in impaired digestion that can lead to intestinal toxemia.

In clinical practice, I have seen literally thousands of patients who have difficulty breaking down foods because of low enzyme levels. As soon as they begin taking supplemental enzymes their digestion improves. They experience less bloating, less belching, and generally feel much better after meals. This not only improves the symptoms, but also helps restore overall digestive health.

There are numerous types of digestive enzymes on the market in all sorts of combinations. But, here's the bottom line: There are two main types of enzymes you need to know about—pancreatic enzymes and plant enzymes. Pancreatic enzymes come from animal sources and are very similar to the enzymes your body makes. These enzymes work in an acidic environment and can be utilized not only for digestion but also can act as anti-inflammatory when taken between meals. In my experience, very few enzymes work as effectively as pancreatic enzymes. I have recommended these products to thousands of patients with excellent results. Bloating, gas, the feeling of fullness and autoimmune-related conditions can all benefit from pancreatic enzymes.

In order for these enzymes to be effective, they should be taken immediately before meals so they can bypass the stomach and travel directly to the duodenum where they can effect digestion. Taking two tablets immediately before a meal and two right after can also be very effective.

I haven't seen the same dramatic results with plant enzymes, although they can be very useful, especially for individuals who are vegetarian. An advantage of plant enzymes is that they work on a broad spectrum of pH's. In other words, they not only work in an acidic environment but they can also work in an alkaline one. This means that they can help digestion in the lower intestinal tract where pH levels are considerably higher than in the stomach and duodenum.

Another benefit of plant enzymes is that they can have broad spectrum effects on carbohydrate digestion. For example, enzymes like cellulose and phytase can help break down various fibers to release minerals and phytochemicals for absorption by the body. Plant enzymes should also be taken immediately prior to meals.

A SPECIAL FORM OF LICORICE

DGL is one of the most under-rated nutritional products in holistic medicine. I find this product invaluable for improving the stomach and duodenal mucosa by increasing the production of mucin. Mucin, as you recall, is the mucous material produced by the stomach and duodenum to protect the lining from the extreme acidic environment. Stress, poor diet, and chemical toxins can impede the production of this mucous, creating an exposed stomach and duodenum lining. This lining then can become victim to the acid which can cause burning, irritation, and even lead to the production of an ulcer.

An extremely effective natural supplement for ulcers is DGL (deglycyrrhizinated licorice). Many researchers have studied DGL for the treatment of gastric and duodenal ulcers. The use of DGL was comparable to standard drug therapy. However, unlike drugs, DGL addresses the underlying factors and promotes true healing by stimulating the body's normal defense mechanisms that prevent ulcer formation. Specifically, DGL improves both the quality and quantity of the protective substances that line the intestinal tract.

DGL is a special extract of licorice from which the glycyrrhizin molecules have been removed, leaving biologically active flavonoids. The value of DGL over other forms of licorice is that it eliminates adverse effects associated with long-term use of very high doses of conventional licorice (including sodium and water retention, high blood pressure, and low potassium levels).

Comparing DGL to other drugs shows just how effective it really is. In 1982, researchers reported in the journal *Gut* that DGL is as effective as cimetidine (Tagamet) for curing gastric ulcers. That same year, the *Lancet* reported DGL to be as effective as ranitidine (Zantac). Researchers also report that licorice root extract stimulates the release of secretin, which in turn has a protective effect on gastric mucosa. The body's production of secretin by such natural agents may play a significant role in their mucosal protective action. In fact, they attribute the anti-ulcer effect of licorice root extract to its unique ability to stimulate the body to release endogenous secretin, which helps to rebuild the stomach's or intestine's protective lining.

Take DGL about 15 minutes before your meals. My recommendation is to take two 380 mg tablets, chewed fully, before each meal for best results.

TABLE 6.2 Comparison Between Antacids, H2- Antagonists And DGL

Therapy	# of Patients	% Healed	% Relapse	Net % Healed
Antacids: 600 mg Al-Mag-OH 5X/day	267	89	16.4	72.6
Cimetidine 200 mg 3X/day	348	93.3	12.9	80.4
DGL 380 mg 3X/day	169	91	8.2	82.8

Irish Med J 78:153-6, 1985

PROBIOTICS

The term probiotic comes from the Greek: *Pro* meaning promoting and *biotic* meaning life. Probiotics are dietary supplements that contain bacteria that are naturally occurring in the human intestine and are beneficial to health. These "good" bacteria colonize in our intestinal tract and play key roles in maintaining nutritional status and immune function, while reducing cancer risk, improving cholesterol metabolism, reducing toxic load, and slowing the aging process. Some might argue that this gives probiotics more credit than they deserve, but research appears to support these very claims.

To understand why probiotics have such an impact on human health we need to realize that a well balanced digestive system is a critical component of a healthy body. Food is broken down in the stomach, digested in the small intestine, then absorbed into the blood stream for utilization throughout the body. An imbalance in good bacteria in the digestive tract can disrupt this process, leading to problems that span from acutely minor to seriously chronic conditions.

How this imbalance leads to disease is something that is only now being understood. Lack of sufficient amounts of good gut bacteria can create an unhealthy gastrointestinal environment which results in impaired digestion and a damaged mucosal gut barrier ("leaky gut") that eventually allows large molecules to enter the blood stream where they can cause autoimmune reactions. It's a domino effect that physicians are starting to look at more closely as the evidence of probiotics' benefit becomes more apparent.

The best way to ensure that you're getting optimal levels of probiotics is to take them as supplements. New research shows that the population of good bacteria in your digestive tract is often not large enough for optimal health. This, in itself, gives us good reason to begin supplementing with probiotics. This can not only help improve digestion but also overall body immune function.

There is, however, a lot of confusion about what kind of probiotics we should take and what counts are best for us. The reality is that probiotics replicate themselves rapidly when they get into the digestive tract. So the key when shopping for a probiotic is to make sure you get one that is stable at room temperature and that offers a delivery system that guarantees that the active bacteria will get to the lower digestive tract where its needed.

Although there are at least four hundred different species of microflora that colonize our gut, the most important strains of healthful bacteria are *Lactobacillus* and *Bifidobacterium*. These bacteria occupy a central role in the gut microflora, thereby enabling them to influence the composition of the microflora to provide health benefits.

But this is only part of the story. In order for probiotics to be effective they need to be live strains that survive the trip to the lower gut. Although probiotics have been available in the marketplace for years, high quality supplements that deliver viable bacteria to the gastrointestinal tract have been very difficult to find.

A recent scientific evaluation of probiotic supplements found that most of them contained 50 percent less of the number of living bacteria that they claimed on their labels. Furthermore, when researchers simulated the acidic stomach environment, they found that, in two popular forms—capsule and liquid—only 10 percent of the living bacteria claimed on the manufacture's label survived the acidic stomach environment.

When looking for a probiotics make sure it is room temperature stable and that the manufacturer guarantees the count that's in the bottle at time of purchase. I often recommend the Acidophilus Pearls by Enzymatic Therapy.

BUILDING A STRONG FOUNDATION

The foundation of all healing is indeed the digestive tract. The fact is, you can't really move forward with detoxification unless this system is in good working order. By following some of the simple tips described you can move towards having a healthy gut in preparation for effective detoxification.

7

CHAPTER SEVEN

Scientific Detoxification

SCIENTIFIC DETOXIFICATION TAKES INTO ACCOUNT ALL that we know about toxic chemicals and our body's natural detoxification system, and creates strategies that can reduce overall toxic body burden and enhance efficient elimination. The important aspect of this concept is that it comes from a scientific point of view and an understanding of how toxicities build up. This provides the avenues necessary for reducing overall exposure and enhancing your body's own ability to get rid of toxic chemicals.

By now you should have a good idea about why you need to detoxify. We're all living in a world where chemical toxicities have been integrated into our own physiology. Studies carried out around the world show us that we are not only retaining chemicals for a short time, some can to linger for decades. This tells us two things:

1. We are exposed to a high level of environmental toxins, and
2. Our body's ability to get rid of them isn't meeting the demands thrown its way.

A good visual of this is the windshield on your car. When it's clean and clear, it's like a toxic free body. Now imagine driving through the snow. Obviously you'll turn on your windshield wipers to remove the falling snowflakes. The snow represents toxins entering your body and the windshield wipers represent your body's own detoxification mechanisms. As the snowfall gets heavier, you increase the speed of the wipers to meet the demands placed on your windshield. But suppose you park outside your house and a huge snowfall drops three feet of snow on your car overnight. When you start the car the next morning, you'll find that the windshield wipers won't work because the load of snow is just too heavy. In order to clear the snow and get the wipers working again, you need to take a broom and sweep the snow off.

Now think of the human body that carries between 400 and 700 toxic chemical and metal residues. Much like that windshield, the body becomes overburdened creating sluggish detoxification systems. What we need to do to lessen this load is two-fold:

- We need to sweep away the excess snow on our windshield. In cleansing terms this means doing a preliminary detoxification program that involves preparing the body and then loosening toxins and helping the body get rid of them.
- Adopt a daily purification and prevention approach, which means making some adjustment to lifestyle that include foods that will minimize chemical exposure and enhance detoxification mechanisms.

THE STEPS

For most people, detoxification means the use of colonics, fasting, lemon juice and honey, and laxatives. Although some of these practices may be beneficial, they fall short of what needs to be done to achieve *whole body cleansing*. The goal of scientific detoxification is to reduce overall body burden by minimizing toxic exposure and increasing the body's ability to detoxify. To accomplish this, we need to make sure that the gastrointestinal tract is in good health, that antioxidant reserves are present for the increased demand, and that Phase I and II detoxification pathways are functioning optimally. Once these steps are followed, then and only then can we achieve successful detoxification.

THE 7 STEPS TO SCIENTIFIC DETOXIFICATION:

- Minimize toxic exposure.
- Optimize bowel health.
- Strengthen antioxidant reserves.
- Improve overall energy production.
- Enhance Phase I and Phase II mechanisms.
- Support toxic metal detoxification.
- Loosen tissue bound toxins.

MINIMIZE TOXIC EXPOSURE

The reason why we need to detoxify is because of the incredible amount of toxic chemicals that our bodies deal with on a daily basis. Over 85,000 chemicals are contained in the thousands of products we use in our everyday lives including carpets, household cleaners, toothpaste, deodorants, moisturizers, perfumes, water, and the chemical additives and pesticides in the food we eat. Minimizing our exposure to these chemicals becomes an important component in any detoxification program.

We reviewed the three entry points in the last chapter—skin, mouth, air passages—and this is a good starting point when we talk about minimizing toxic exposure. Studies have shown that the air inside of our homes is more toxic than the air outdoors. This sometimes comes as a shock to people because we are conditioned to think that only outdoor air is contaminated. But the reality is that the air inside our homes is laced with toxic fumes coming from carpeting, paint, household cleaning products, and air conditioners. So our first step is to minimize this exposure by dealing with the entry points.

STEPS TO MINIMIZE TOXIC EXPOSURE:

REDUCE THE USE OF TOXIC HOUSEHOLD CLEANING PRODUCTS. There are a number of biodegradable toxin free cleaning agents that are not only better for the environment outside, but also for the environment inside your house.

REDUCE THE USE OF TOXIC BEAUTY PRODUCTS. Start using soaps that are free of chemical additives, antiperspirants that are free of aluminum, toothpastes and moisturizers with only natural ingredients. Look for them at your local health food store.

BECOME AWARE OF THE FOODS YOU CONSUME. Begin eating organic produce that is free of pesticides and herbicides—the cost is not much different. If you can't get organic, make sure you wash all of your vegetables with natural cleaning solutions and peel your fruit.

If you are going to eat meat, BEGIN SHIFTING TO ORGANICALLY-GROWN MEAT FREE OF HORMONES AND CHEMICAL ADDITIVES. Be aware of the fish you consume and stay away from farm-raised salmon that have high PCB counts.

GET A GOOD AIR FILTER to reduce the amount of toxins that are re-circulated throughout your home. Remember the air in your home is full of toxic chemicals, getting rid of them will reduce your overall exposure.

MAKE SURE THE WATER YOU DRINK IS PURIFIED. Add a filtration system to your shower head to make sure bathing water is clean and toxic free. Remember your skin is an organ and a highly absorbable one at that.

These steps are important in your quest for optimal health. It's not easy to change old habits but, if you do, you'll find yourself feeling better, looking better, and living better.

OPTIMIZE BOWEL HEALTH

Although we discussed digestion in great detail in Chapter 6, let's do a quick review and focus on some important points as they relate to detoxification. As I mentioned, the gastrointestinal tract plays a pivotal role in detoxification and also in maintaining a healthy immune system. Body healing can't progress until the digestive tract is healed.

Key steps for creating a healthy gastrointestinal tract:

- Remove pathogenic organisms.
- Support the digestive process by supplementing with pancreatic enzymes.

- Replenish good bacteria in the intestinal tract with live, active probiotics.
- Support mucin production with DGL.
- Ensure sufficient fiber consumption to normalize bowel health.

On the surface, this sounds like a lot of work, but it's not—and the benefits far outweigh the effort. Patients become generally healthier as they optimize digestive health by utilizing these five key steps. Let's look at these steps in more detail:

1. If you've been diagnosed with yeast or other invasive organisms, the first step is to remove these pathogenic organisms. The most well-researched remedies for this job are oregano oil (*Origanum vulgare*) and thyme (*Thymus vulgaris*) which both contain carvacrol and thymol, two compounds that have powerful anti-microbial effects with an affinity for yeast. Along with these herbs, consider using a good soluble-insoluble fiber supplement to bind the toxins released from the destruction of these micro-organisms. Both soluble and insoluble fibers are important. I'll address that a little later in this chapter.

2. Supporting digestive processes with pancreatic enzymes is a very effective way of improving digestion. Highly processed, chemically-filled foods, combined with everyday stress, can shut down digestion. But digestive enzymes, especially pancreatic enzymes, closely resemble human enzymes and can greatly facilitate the digestive process. If you have a feeling a fullness, bloating and gas, and occasional acid moving up into your esophagus, you are a prime candidate for pancreatic enzyme. These are very fast acting enzymes, so take two tablets immediately before meals and you should see results very quickly.

3. Probiotics have now been shown to collectively perform functions that are essential for our health. Research shows that the population of friendly bacteria in our gastrointestinal tracts isn't large enough for optimal health. This often results in the rise of harmful bacteria, which causes an imbalance. This negatively effects overall digestive function.

Supplementing with probiotics is an essential step in optimizing bowel health.

When you look for a probiotic, keep a number of things in mind. Make sure the product has a true delivery system which guarantees that a certain amount of live bugs get to the intestine. Also look for a room temperature culture that doesn't need to be refrigerated. This helps ensure that what the label says is what you'll actually get. Lastly, the most common bugs are *Lactobacillus acidophilus* and *Bifidobacterium longum*; take about 2 billion of these daily to ensure a healthy digestive tract.

4. There is a component in the stomach and the gastrointestinal tract that plays a big role protecting the intestinal lining. Produced by mucous cells, mucin is a viscous liquid that not only protects the integrity of the intestinal cells but also protects them from the acidic environment of the stomach. The pH of the stomach during digestion is around 1.2, which is enough to dissolve metal. Mucin allows the lining to withstand such acidity.

   To improve the quality and quantity of mucin, DGL is probably the best natural ingredient available. In clinical studies, this amazing product benefits people with ulcers and gastroesophageal reflux (GERD) by improving the quality and quantity of mucin, increasing the life-span of intestinal cells, and improving mucosal blood flow. To make DGL work for you, chew two tablets 15 minutes before meals and as needed between meals. Because it must be chewed, there are different flavors available to make it easier for people to comply.

5. The last thing you need to do to optimize bowel health is to ensure that you are getting enough dietary fiber in your diet. Dietary fiber is essential to normalize bowel transit time, blood sugar levels, and blood cholesterol levels. It also supports detoxification mechanisms. When looking for a detoxification kit make sure it contains a high quality combination of both soluble and insoluble fiber. Psyllium, pectin, oat bran, guar gum, and marshmallow root are the combinations I often

recommend. This gives you a great blend of both soluble and insoluble fibers, which each have specific functions for detoxification benefits.

Soluble fiber is important because it binds bile as it enters the intestine from the liver and gallbladder. Remember bile carries all of the toxic compounds that are released during detoxification. Fiber grabs this toxin-filled bile and holds onto it until the body can eliminate it. Insoluble fiber helps the body eliminate toxins held in the colon by gently scrubbing the intestinal walls. This helps to carry pathogenic micro-organisms and debris out of the body.

STRENGTHEN ANTIOXIDANT RESERVES

As we learned in Chapter 5, an active Phase I pathway neutralizes a lot of toxins but also creates free radicals. These free radicals are usually handled by Phase II, but when Phase II isn't working up to par, free radicals accumulate and begin to use up your supply of glutathione. Depleting glutathione reserves is very serious and creates a vulnerable situation in the body.

To get a better picture of what happens, let's take a closer look at free radicals and antioxidants. The action of free radicals is similar to slicing an apple in half and watching the exposed white flesh turn brown. If you take another apple and slice it in half, but this time squeeze lemon juice on it, it doesn't brown because the lemon juice is the antioxidant that prevents discoloration. The absence of glutathione in the body creates cell damage, much like the apple without the lemon.

Since we don't want this cellular damage to occur, we need to make sure we have plenty of antioxidants to help combat the growing levels of free radicals created during Phase I. There are a number of antioxidants that can help. These include milk thistle (*Silybum marianum*), vitamins C and E, and selenium. I would also recommend N-Acetyl-Cysteine (NAC), which helps build new glutathione, and resveratrol, a powerful new antioxidant with lots of benefits.

ENHANCE OVER ALL ENERGY PRODUCTION

An important aspect of detoxification is that it is energy dependent and always active. In fact, detoxification is the biggest user of energy outside the brain. The detoxification pathways need a continuous supply of ATP. As we've seen, ATP is produced in the energy factories of the cells called mitochondria. The process involves the mitochondria taking oxygen and sugar and, through a complex network of reactions, creating ATP. But in order for this reaction to run smoothly, an important cofactor called coenzyme Q10 (CoQ10) is essential.

CoQ10 is naturally produced in the body but age, medications, and dietary habits may interfere with the amount of CoQ10 the body makes. Supplementing with 100 to 200 mg of CoQ10 per day is beneficial because it will enhance overall energy production.

But here is the catch: Very little of the CoQ10 on the market is actually absorbed into cells where it can do its work. So when you look for a supplement, look for a high quality, well-studied CoQ10 supplement that can be delivered to desired sites. To date there is only one CoQ10 supplement—Vitaline CoQ10—that is clinically proven to cross cell membranes and reach the mitochondria where it improves cellular energy production. Look for the Vitaline CoQ10 ingredient on the label.

ENHANCE PHASE I AND PHASE II MECHANISMS IN THE LIVER

As I've mentioned, the liver is the most important organ for detoxification. Improving antioxidant status, energy production, and even bowel function supports the liver in its daily detoxification work. Enhancing its Phase I and Phase II mechanisms are at the center of any scientific detoxification program.

BOTANICAL MEDICINES

An important way of supporting the detoxification pathways is to utilize botanical medicines that have some scientific evidence backing their efficacy. There a number of different phytomedicines that fit these criteria and that should be incorporated in supporting these pathways. They include milk thistle (*Silybum marianum*), turmeric (*Curcuma longa*), artichoke extract (*Cynara scolymus*) and dandelion root (*Taraxacum officinale*). Let's take a closer look.

Milk thistle is one of the best known botanicals for liver conditions. It has been used by holistically-oriented physicians, herbalists, and nutritionists for decades with great success. There is even a fair amount of research validating some of the physiological benefits of this impressive botanical medicine.

The active component in milk thistle, *silymarin*, contains four flavolignans. The most researched, *silybin*, has powerful antioxidant properties specific to the liver. It is effective in controlling the free radicals produced during Phase I detoxification. Silymarin can also help regenerate liver cells, enhance the liver's ability to destroy foreign organisms, and increase glutathione levels.

Milk thistle's antioxidant properties are due to the fact that it can actually increase glutathione levels. Glutathione, as we've talked about earlier, is the key antioxidant for the liver, as well as throughout the entire body. Increasing levels of glutathione in the liver by utilizing both botanical and nutritional means is an extremely important technique in enhancing detoxification. Many of the problems of detoxification stem from low glutathione stores. Glutathione is also the most important chelator (binder) of toxic metals in the body.

This herb also helps stimulate protein synthesis in the liver. What this ultimately means is that it helps regenerate liver cells. The liver is an organ in the body that regenerates itself; milk thistle facilitates that process. This botanical also activates white blood cells known as Kuffer cells. Kuffer cells are macrophages which help engulf bad bacteria and viruses within the liver.

One of the problems with most milk thistle supplements is that they are poorly absorbed. Very few people know this and are under the mistaken impression that when you purchase an ingredient or when that ingredient is part of a product that it gets into the blood and goes where it is suppose to. This is a good way of thinking; unfortunately botanicals and other nutritional products don't always behave that way. In fact, studies show that when regular milk thistle was compared to a milk thistle bound to phosphatidyl choline (PC). The PC bound supplement was absorbed seven times as effectively. In other words, even though the starting dosage was exactly the same, the PC-bound milk thistle was absorbed 700 percent more efficiently than a regular milk thistle supplement of the same dosage. When looking at whole body detoxification kits make sure the milk thistle is bound to phosphatidylcholine, forming a new complex (phytosome) that increases milk thistle's absorption by seven times.

Turmeric has been one of my favorite botanical medicines because of its many useful applications. Because of its active compound, curcumin, this Indian spice has been shown to possess possible anti-inflammatory properties as well as liver support functions. Some animal studies have shown *curcuma longa* to not only slow down and inhibit certain Phase I enzymes but also enhance Phase II reactions by inducing glutathione S-transferase activity. This has some important applications in detoxification reactions. For example, overexposure to toxins speeds up Phase I reactions but has no effect on Phase II conjugation reactions. This leads to an overabundance of Phase I by-products which become extremely reactive and damaging. Curcumin can bring balance by slowing down Phase I, thus allowing Phase II to catch up and reduce the amount of intermediate products that could cause havoc to liver cells. Curcumin may also reduce the incidence of gallstones, another possible plus for detoxification reactions.

Artichoke has a long history of use for liver support. Its active ingredients include cynarin, cynardoside (luteolin-7-O-glycoside) and chlorogenic acid, all of which support liver function. Studies point out that these ingredients help in the secretion of bile (choleresis). As we've seen, bile is an important component in detoxification since it is the carrier that moves all final Phase II packaged toxins out of the liver. Its production and movement are critical to the process of detoxification. Artichoke supports and enhances this overall process.

Another important function of artichoke is its role as an anti-oxidant. Free radicals are produced during detoxification, so antioxidants are an important safeguard against them. Artichoke also has been established as a hepato-protective herb. This means that it can help protect the liver from a variety of toxins.

Dandelion root is another common botanical used in many detoxification formulas. Its principal uses for detoxification lie in its affect on the gallbladder and kidneys. Studies show that dandelion's active ingredient increases bile production and flow to the gallbladder, exerting a direct effect on the organ and causing the contraction and release of stored bile (cholagogue). Again, bile movement is important because it gets toxins out of the liver and into the digestive tract for quick elimination.

Other research has found that dandelion root is an excellent diuretic that does not compromise potassium. Many diuretics lower potassium levels; dandelion root stimulates diuresis and supplies potassium. The overall benefit is that, since the kidneys play an important role in detoxification (removal of steroidal hormones, etc.), enhancing their function helps the body remove toxins.

IMPORTANT NUTRIENTS

One of the most important things to remember is that we are exposed to chemical toxins 24 hours a day, 365 days a year. What this illustrates is that, even though it is important to cleanse two to three times per year, we should also be taking nutritional support as part of a daily regimen. This includes a number of nutritional ingredients that help support active Phase I and Phase II detoxification pathways. Table 7.1 and 7.2 summarize the most important nutritional ingredients and their role in detoxification activities. When looking for a supplement to support daily detoxification requirements make sure it contains some of the ingredients listed in these two tables.

TABLE 7.1 Nutritional ingredients supporting Phase I detoxification pathway

Phase I Nutritional Support	
Antioxidant	Detoxification Activities
Reduced Glutathione (GSH)	Highest concentration in the liver, also in white blood cells. Prevents formation of free radical chain reactions and vital for regeneration of other antioxidants. Levels decline with age and with excess free radical formation.
N-Acetyl-L-Cysteine (NAC)	Precursor of glutathione, promotes healthy detoxification and the elimination of intestinal endotoxins.
CoQ10	Important component of energy production.
Vitamin C	Plays a role in liver's detoxification activities, especially the detoxification of mercury.
Vitamin E	Protects cell membranes from free radical damage.
Selenium	Important in liver's ability to eliminate arsenic. Along with vitamin C, supports glutathione production.
Quercetin	Bioflavonoid found in green tea, red cabbage, tomatoes, cherries, and grapes. Excellent antioxidant that also enhances liver enzyme detoxification mechanisms.

TABLE 7.2 Nutritional ingredients supporting Phase II detoxification pathways

Phase II Nutritional Support	
Conjugating Agents	Detoxification Activities
Calcium D-glucarate (CDG)	Precursor of glucarolactone (GL), which inhibits B-glucuronidase. CDG supplementation increases net elimination of toxins and steroid hormones via Phase II.
Glutathione (GSH)	Adequate amounts of GSH result in increased elimination of toxins and steroid hormones.
N-Acetyl-L-Cysteine (NAC)	Supports glutathione production, which will enhance the elimination of drugs, neurotransmitters, steroids, intestinal toxins, and heavy metals.
Vitamin B6	Used in reducing the levels of homocysteine, a very toxic free radical linked to heart disease.
Vitamin B12 / Folic Acid	Important cofactor in methylation reactions (both exogenous and endogenous compounds).
Glycine, Taurine Glutamine	Utilized in amino acid conjugation reactions such as detoxification of ammonia.
Alpha-Lipoic Acid	Also called thioctic acid, it is a universal antioxidant because it is soluble in both fat and water. A powerful antioxidant that can neutralize all free radicals and can also enhance the antioxidant functions of Vitamins C and E, and glutathione.

SUPPORT TOXIC METAL DETOXIFICATION

Heavy metals are present in almost every human being on the planet. Exposure comes from burning of fossil fuels, fish consumption, dental amalgam fillings, vaccines, paint, and a number of other sources (see table 7.3).

TABLE 7.3 Toxic metals and their toxic effects

Toxic Metal	Toxicities/Accumulation	Sources
Cadmium	Peripheral artery disease Endothelium damage (atherosclerosis end result) Accumulates in the kidneys	Shellfish Bottom fish Fossil fuels
Mercury (Hg)	Neurological: Reduces nerve conduction, inhibits serotonin and dopamine (depression, Parkinson's) Renal Cardiovascular Immunological: Increases antibiotic resistance Elemental Hg forms methyl-mercury (95% absorbable)	Predatory fish / tuna Inhalation Amalgams
Lead	Hematological: Interferes with heme production (carries oxygen) Neurological: Blood-brain barrier GI effects: Spasms around smooth muscle Renal effects	Paint Gasoline Lipstick Water

The best way of reducing toxic metals is to ensure optimal glutathione levels in the body. This special antioxidant has been shown to chelate both lead and cadmium from the bloodstream and reduce mercury levels. By ensuring optimum levels of glutathione, you are also going a long way in supporting toxic metal elimination.

A few ways of ensuring optimum levels of glutathione are through taking milk thistle, NAC, and alpha lipoic acid. Another method of increasing glutathione levels directly is by taking a product known as recancostat. Recancostat is a patented nutritional formula consisting of anthocyans, L-cysteine, and most importantly, reduced glutathione.

This is the only form of supplemental glutathione clinically shown to get into the blood. It is used by doctors in Europe and is now available in North America.

SUMMARY

Familiarizing yourself with what needs to be done to support detoxification is just the first step in the science of detoxification. The next step is knowing when and how to take the recommended nutrients. In the past, detoxification programs involved taking a bag of products for seven to 14 days and repeating the process two to three times a year. The new paradigm is a scientifically formulated detoxification program you do three times a year. But, in addition, you also need to carry out daily purification and prevention strategies for long term effects. See Chapter 12, *Putting it all Together*.

8

Moving Toxins Out of Tissues

UP TO THIS POINT, OUR DISCUSSION has focused on the toxicities found in the human body and what effect they may be having. By now you should be starting to realize what may be contributing to the chronic conditions that are so prevalent in our society. You should also be gaining some insight into why so many children are falling prey to so many new diseases. It's obvious that when you disrupt normal physiology in the human body with toxic chemicals, health problems result.

SO, WHAT NOW?

In order for us to create the internal (body) environment that supports the healing process we must eliminate the obstacles to cure. This means creating an environment where the body can function optimally. The goals of this process include improving digestion, improving antioxidant status, optimizing energy production, and most importantly, reducing total body burden.

Body burden, as we've learned, is the total amount of toxins present in the body at any given time. It is not a number we can ever truly measure but it is something we can use to define what it is we are trying to lower. For example, chemicals are stored in body fat, in bones, and in a number of other tissues. It would be a very costly and arduous to calculate how much and what kind of chemicals are stored.

THE PROBLEM WITH PRESCRIPTIONS

Although prescription and over-the-counter (OTC) drugs have helped countless individuals with symptomatic relief, one must ask if these drugs are overused and what impact that overuse my have on our bodies and our environment. According to a CNN report, when people take their prescription, some of the drug residue makes its way into municipal drinking water and even in some bottled water. What this is telling us is that we are being saturated with these medications whether we are prescribed them or not. And although these medications may help with symptoms they don't seem to be helping solve our health problems. As a culture, we need to look beyond symptom relief, which will in turn reduce our usage of the countless drugs being prescribed and taken over the counter.

What we can do, however, is calculate easily tested toxic pollutants to get some idea of body burden. A number of laboratories in the United States offer testing for toxic metals, pesticides, PCB's, dioxins, and other useful indicators of the body's toxic load (body burden).

We can also test the liver to understand how efficiently the detoxification pathways are working. This also gives us some valuable information about our body burden. In other words, if the body's detoxification pathways are compromised, that means lower levels of these toxins are being eliminated, giving us a higher body burden.

MOVING TOXINS

Moving toxins out of the tissues is what this chapter is all about. When people think of detoxification, they think of certain products that will supposedly help the body get rid of circulating chemicals. But this isn't the whole story. We not only need to help the body get rid of circulating toxins, we need to get rid of stored toxins as well. In order to accomplish this task, we'll need to loosen the toxins that are bound to tissues. This is similar to removing a stubborn stain from your favorite shirt. Before placing the shirt in the washer, you spray it with a spot remover.

This process loosens the stain, which allows your laundry detergent to easily remove it from the item.

Moving toxins out of tissues is a similar process. You need to first loosen the chemicals and then clean them up and remove them from the body. Obviously, the area that contains the greatest amount of stored chemicals is your adipose tissue. This includes the fat distributed throughout the body, including the brain. These tissues contain toxic chemicals for two reasons:

- Because the body wasn't able to eliminate enough of them.
- Most chemicals are fat soluble.

In order for us to achieve true detoxification we need to move toxins out of these tissues. Obviously, we can't use a spot remover, so we need to use other techniques that will give us the required results. Science has shown that a number of methodologies work well in loosening these toxins and bringing them into the open so our detoxification mechanisms can remove them from our bodies.

THE PROCESS

The process of removing chemical toxins from tissues has to be well organized to avoid possible side effects. As we've seen in Chapter 7, there are a number of things that you need to do to have success:

- Reduce overall exposure and enhance body physiology through diet.
- Enhance antioxidant status.
- Loosen stored toxins.
- Enhance Phase I and Phase II detoxification mechanisms.
- Improve gastrointestinal health so toxins can be safely eliminated out of the body.

In this chapter, we are going to focus on loosening stored toxins. This is an important aspect of detoxification yet, when done incorrectly, it can be the most damaging. Let me explain. When you begin to loosen chemical toxins like pesticides and toxic metals from adipose tissues, these compounds enter the blood stream. Once in circulation—and depending on their concentrations—these chemicals can be extremely toxic. They can cause lots of damage as is usually observed with patients who are constantly fasting.

The proper way of loosening toxins from body tissues is to make sure that your body's elimination system is ready for the challenge. This involves making sure glutathione levels are healthy, and that the liver and gastrointestinal tract are both functioning optimally. Last but not least, you want to make sure that your diet supports detoxification pathways.

TOXINS ARE STORED

One of the most important things to understand about chemical toxins is that there are so many of them that your body just can't get rid of them efficiently. A portion of these chemicals end up being incorporated into bodily tissue, where they can stay for years—even decades. This has been proven in many different studies including the National Human Adipose Tissue Survey (NHATS).

NHATS was a study conducted by the EPA to analyze the amount of toxic chemicals found in human adipose tissues. The goal was to investigate the presence of toxic chemicals in the environment and its direct effect on our bodies. During the eleven year period (1976-1987), pathologists and medical examiners from dozens of metropolitan areas collected and analyzed samples of adipose tissue specimens for the presence of chemicals. The results were shocking. One hundred percent of all samples contained chemical toxins. They found pesticides, PCBs, dioxins, furans, OCDD (dioxins found in dairy and meat products), volatile organic compounds, semivolatile organic compounds, styrene, 1,4-dichlorobenzene, and xylene.

It should be noted that these chemical were not eliminated by the body as they should have been. So the question is, why didn't the body eliminate them, why are they still present, and what can we do about it?

The reason we find so many chemicals stored in the body is because our detoxification system just can't keep up with the level of exposure. Remember, we create all sorts of endogenous toxins that our bodies are constantly cleaning up. Add to that the enormous amount

TABLE 8.1 National Human Adipose Survey

Compound	Frequency
Styrene	100%
1,4-dichlorobenzene	100%
Xylene	100%
OCDD (dioxin)	100%
Ethylphenol	100%
9 other chemicals*	90-98%
PCBs	83%

of exogenous toxins and we have the "several feet of snow" analogy. Our system can't deal with the build up so the body protects itself by pulling them out of circulation and storing them in adipose tissue and bones. The problem is that, eventually, something occurs to cause the release of these toxins.

HOW TO RELEASE TOXINS

An important aspect of scientific detoxification is the release of toxins that are bound to body tissues. We've extensively discussed the fact that toxins are all around us and that our bodies are absorbing them. To some degree, we've begun discussing how to reduce exposure and improve our body's ability to get rid of these toxins. But how exactly do we loosen bound toxins?

Loosening toxins again requires an understanding of not only the methodologies of the process but also the preparation of the detoxification system. As we mentioned earlier, once toxins are released they enter the blood stream, causing all sorts of damage. The only way we can prevent this damage is if we control the release and prepare the body to be able to deal with the tidal wave of toxins.

The majority of toxins stored in the body are found in adipose tissue or other fat-based tissues (nerve tissues included). One of the functions of the detoxification system in the liver is to render these toxins water soluble so they become removable. Knowing this fact, the easiest and most cost effective way of loosening these toxins from fat tissue is to dissolve the fat. This can be accomplished in a number of ways:

- Exercise and weight loss.
- Saunas, including infrared.
- Fasting.
- Chemical binding agents.

The first three methods have one thing in common; they cause the release of chemicals from adipose tissue by moving the tissue and/or breaking down the tissue. This, in turn, releases the chemicals and raises blood levels. The fourth method uses chelating agents to bind specific types of toxins. For example, DMSA (2,3-dimercaptosuccinic acid) is used to bind mercury. It has the ability to enter cells of all tissues and organs and remove the heavy metal. Although DMSA is specific and doesn't have broad spectrum application, it does loosen mercury and other toxic metals from adipose and other tissues. We are actually doing that to some degree everyday—we just aren't aware of it. When you go for that long walk, that hike, that bike ride; when you lift those weights at the gym or putter in your garden, you are loosening up some toxins. Obviously, the more intensely you do these activities, the more toxins are released.

METHODOLOGIES

EXERCISE: If there is one aspect of lifestyle known to have tremendous health benefits, its exercise. We've heard the positives from our favorite athletes and health gurus, and even by just watching the latest installment of the popular television show The Biggest Loser. But do we really know why it's so good for us? In my experience, the answer is no! Almost every patient I have seen in the last 20 years is in agreement that exercise will make them healthier but they don't know the full story of how. I often share the importance of exercise with my patients and friends who don't exercise. It seems that when people truly understand the underlying principles of its benefits they begin to include exercise in their daily routines. These benefits include:

- Increasing lung capacity and improving cardiovascular function.
- Improving the movement lymph through the lymphatic system.
- Triggering the release of a number of compounds that can help repair tissues and keep you young.
- Helping reduce overall body fat, which helps the body release stored toxins.

Improving lung capacity and cardiovascular function has long been known as a benefit of exercise. Do you remember running your first mile in high school and how tired you were at the finish line? Did you notice that, as you kept running week in and week out, it got progressively easier. That's because you were increasing your lung capacity and improving cardiovascular function. Your body was adapting to the stress and improving certain aspects of your physiology to accomplish the task.

An area of benefit that many of us don't understand is the lymphatic system. The lymphatic system is a pipe system (like the circulatory system) that carries lymph from the interstitium into the lymph nodes and then back into the circulatory system. The 100 trillion cells in your body have spaces between them; this space makes up approximately one-sixth of your body volume and is called the interstitium. The interstitial fluid is made from cells dumping their fluids and metabolic wastes into the space. Much of this debris gets picked up by tiny blood vessels; another chunk gets picked up by the lymphatic vessels (which make up the lymphatic system). This fluid that enters the lymphatic system becomes what is known as lymph.

Once this fluid enters the lymphatic vessels, it is taken to a nearby lymphatic node where it is filtered. If the node, which is really like an investigation factory, finds something wrong with the fluid (virus, cancer, toxic chemical), the lymph node swells up as it starts attracting white blood cells in order to deal with the problem. If, on the other hand, everything is fine the lymph fluid continues and eventually gets dumped into the blood circulation system via the subclavian veins.

One of the biggest differences between the cardiovascular system and the lymphatic system is that the lymphatic system doesn't have a pump like the heart. Instead the fluid movement is strictly dependent on the smooth muscles lining the lymph vessels. Exercise can stimulate this smooth muscle lining and improve overall lymphatic movement; an important aspect of helping to move toxins out of cells. Exercise also helps lymph fluids circulate throughout the body, which removes toxins and other harmful materials.

Another important aspect of exercise is that a number of compounds are released during stressful body movements. These chemicals are not just endorphins but other possible mediators that can help repair body tissues and prevent premature aging. Endorphins have been talked about in the past because they are the "make you feel good" chemicals. We know that the release of these chemicals can make you feel better and actually improve overall performance.

What this doesn't explain is why exercise has been linked to a reduction in heart disease, an improvement in blood sugar regulation, an enhancement in immune function and an overall improvement in general well-being. Why does exercise have so many benefits? The answer to this question may lie in something we've already discussed, the epigenome. Could exercise have a positive impact on the epigenome, turning off genes that have negative health effects and improving so many health parameters? This is definitely a possibility. But, until science can fully answer this question, it's important to keep right on exercising.

Last but not least, exercise can help you lose weight and maintain your physical shape. How many people do you know that begin an exercise program to lose weight? Lots of them! But what they haven't known is that losing weight, more specifically losing fat, results in the release of chemical toxins. This is both useful and also very counter productive if you don't take all the right precautions.

Let me tell you about a study that was done in 2004 on a group of individuals following a weight loss program. The study followed 64 people who, for three months, followed a specific diet and exercise regime. Weight measurements were taken every two weeks, fat loss was measured, as were pesticide levels and active thyroid hormone (T3). During the course of the study, as the women lost more and more adipose tissue, the pesticide level in their blood stream continually rose. This makes sense since toxins are stored in fat and, as we exercise and lose fat, these chemicals are released into the blood stream. But here is the interesting thing—as their pesticide count went up, production of T3 from the thyroid went down. This, in turn, slowed down their metabolic rates and affected further weight loss. Although this hasn't been confirmed, it could be the reason so many people going through weight loss programs often plateau and can't lose any further weight. Perhaps, something that all weight loss programs should consider is adding a good detoxification program along with every weight loss system.

SAUNAS

One of the basic steps of detoxification is promoting the release of lipophilic (fat soluble) toxins from the fat cells of the body. There are those who believe this can be done with heat and the process is known as heat depuration. The idea behind this technique is just like putting butter in a hot pan; the butter melts. This same type of concept is supposed to happen to adipose tissue in the body during heat depuration. The proponents, and there are many, that use a sauna for this technique claim that utilizing infrared is the better approach for two reasons. First, the temperature doesn't get as hot as the air sauna's (169-200 degree F) and second, the infrared rays penetrate deeper into the skin getting to the fat tissues. This vibrates adipose cells and loosens bound toxins.

Although many in the mainstream medical world may claim that sauna's have not been scientifically studied, there is enough history to claim that they are an effective way of loosening bound toxins. With their popularity growing and the costs going down, infrared saunas are now available at a number of department outlets for purchase. This is an excellent adjunct to a detoxification program because you can start slowly and gradually increase your time as you begin to get rid of toxic chemicals.

My recommendation is always to begin with 15 minute sessions, ensuring proper hydration throughout the process. As you become more accustomed and educated to the use of the sauna, you can increase your exposure.

Once again, when using a sauna, make sure you check with your doctor, especially if your blood pressure is elevated. Always have proper hydration while in the sauna and make sure you have plenty of detoxification support in order to bind the chemicals as they are being emitted from your fat tissues.

NUTRIENTS AND CHELATION

There are a few products that have been used to loosen certain toxic chemicals bound to tissues. Most of these products should be used under the supervision of a physician because dosages need to be carefully monitored depending on individual variability. Also, some of these products can only be administered intravenously because their absorption through the gut wall is limited.

The word chelation or chelator is often used to describe these types of products. Chelation comes the Greek word "*chele*" meaning claw; a claw grabs things, a chelator also grabs things. Chelation is a process where certain agents are used to detoxify the body of various toxic chemicals like mercury, cadmium, lead, and arsenic. The chelation molecule has the ability to make these toxins soluble in blood and therefore allows them to be eliminated out of the body. Chelation therapy is also used by some physicians in an attempt to treat autism.

EDTA: Ethylenediamine tetra-acetic acid (EDTA) has been used in medicine for decades. It is a substance with an ability to bind various metals, including toxic metals, and make them soluble in blood. This solubility allows these toxic metals to be eliminated through the kidneys in the urine.

EDTA has to be intravenously administered since the molecule is very poorly absorbed. If someone wants this type of treatment, it must be administered by a physician trained in chelation protocols. There are a number of things an individual going through a chelation program needs to be tested for. An important parameter to measure is whether or not the kidneys are properly functioning. Since EDTA chelation allows the excretion of metals through the kidneys, they need to be functioning optimally to be able to take on the extra work. Also, people going through EDTA chelation often develop hypoglycemia (low blood sugar) during treatment so this needs to be monitored. If you are interested in chelation therapy for loosening toxic metals from tissues, make sure you visit a physician and become thoroughly educated about the process.

DMSA: It has long been recognized that sulfur-containing compounds have the ability to chelate heavy metals. There are a number of naturally-occurring sulfur-containing compounds—and some even made within the body—which perform this task. These include N-acetyl cysteine (NAC), alpha-lipoic acid, S-adenysyl methionine (SAMe), and glutathione (GSH).

DMSA does not occur naturally in the human body, nor is it a constituent of food. However, it has been studied for over 40 years as an effective oral chelator of toxic metals. Initial studies took place in the People's Republic of China, Japan, and Russia, and then spread to Europe and the USA. DMSA (2,3-Dimercaptosuccinic acid) is FDA approved and something I have used extensively, especially during challenge testing (more about that later). It is given orally to treat mercury poisoning. This ingredient has the ability to enter cells and organ systems, grab mercury, and eliminate it in the urine via the kidneys. DMSA can also be used to chelate other toxic metals like lead, cadmium, and arsenic. Again, it needs to be administered by a trained physician but the results are very good.

DMSA TREATMENT IN MERCURY TOXICITY

In the United States, DMSA was first reported to promote mercury excretion without many side effects in 1975. Since that time, numerous animal and human studies have shown DMSA administration increases urinary mercury excretion and reduces blood and tissue mercury concentration. In a comparison study of chelating agents, 11 construction workers with acute mercury poisoning were treated with either DMSA or N-acetyl-D, L-penicillamine (NAP, a toxic metal binder). DMSA treatment resulted in greater urinary excretion of mercury than NAP. One of the problems with mercury is that it can easily get into the brain, which causes all sorts of problems. Animal studies on DMSA's ability to reduce brain mercury levels have shown this product to be the most efficient chelator of brain mercury.

In another animal study, DMSA was given four days after mercury injection in mice, and continued for eight days. DMSA removed two-thirds of the brain mercury deposits, NAP removed approximately one-half, while DMPs did not remove significant amounts of mercury from the brain. DMP (2,3-dimercaptopropane-1-Sulphonate) is another binding agent that has been shown to grab toxic metals stored in tissues. However, I do not use DMPs since it is not FDA approved and because of the possibilities of side effects.

MERCURY DIAGNOSTIC AND TREATMENT PROTOCOL

An effective way to evaluate mercury toxicity quantitatively is to determine the amount of mercury excreted in the urine after a challenge dose of DMSA. Let me explain: The way we measure mercury levels is to test the toxic metal in the urine. The body is constantly trying to detoxify toxic metals through Phase II conjugation reactions (glutathione conjugation being the main one). Once it goes through Phase II, it enters the blood and is eliminated via the urine. But, if you haven't been exposed to mercury for a long time, the blood levels may be low and a test of the urine is not going to show much mercury. This however, doesn't mean you don't have a high body burden of mercury; it may simply be stored in the tissues.

When I perform toxic metal testing in my clinic, one of the things I do is first test the urine without a challenge. Once that is done and the patient has collected the day's urine sample, we make them collect another sample, but this time they will take DMSA beforehand. The DMSA will loosen mercury and other toxic metals from tissues which will end up in the urine sample. In many cases we get little toxic metal showing up in the baseline test but a lot of toxic metal showing up in the challenge test. This gives us valuable information about the storage of these metals in body tissues.

LEAD TOXICITY

DMSA has been used for lead poisoning since the 1950s. In recent studies DMSA has been shown to be a safe and effective chelator of lead, reducing blood levels significantly. In the present study, regular dosage reduced lead blood levels by 36 percent while at much higher dosages blood lead levels were reduced by nearly 73 percent. Clinical symptoms and biochemical indices of lead toxicity also improved.

DOSAGE

The dosage of DMSA for mercury toxicity or other toxic metals is not clear. Some physicians have given dosages as high as 30 mg/kg of body weight. This dosage means that an individual weighing 110 pounds (50 kg) would take approximately 1,500 mg of DMSA per day (50 multiplied by 30 mg).

A protocol I often use is 500 mg every other day on an empty stomach for about six weeks. Some patients may be sensitive to DMSA, so lowering the dosage can be helpful. Other dosing includes taking 10mg/kg of body weight taken in divided doses for three days. The patient then stops for 14 days before starting again for three days for a total of five to 10 treatment cycles. Obviously more studies need to be done to figure out what the optimal dosages actually are; however, because of the safety record, more physicians have had a good grasp on DMSA's dosing parameters.

ADJUNCT NUTRITIONALS

During this DMSA process, utilizing hydrolyzed whey protein may also be of benefit because it contains high amounts of cysteine residues. Cysteine is the rate-limiting step in glutathione production. Taking 500 mg of NAC (N-acetylcysteine) three times per day can also be helpful.

Remember NAC is important in regenerating glutathione, the body's natural toxic metal chelator.

When taking any chelating product it is always a good idea to take a multi-mineral supplement. DMSA, EDTA and other chelation substances not only chelate toxic metals, they can also chelate good minerals like zinc and magnesium. Supplementing ensures that optimal levels are always present.

FINAL THOUGHTS

Detoxification doesn't simply mean taking some supplements and hoping that everything goes away. It involves reducing exposure and actually moving stored toxins out of tissues and into the blood where the liver and other detoxification organs can do their job and eliminate these toxic chemicals. There are a number of methods that can move toxins from adipose tissue into the circulation. Exercise, saunas, and carefully selected physician prescribed substances can all be effective in moving stored toxins for detoxification.

CHAPTER NINE

Fiber And The Every Day Detoxification Diet

THE WORD DETOXIFICATION HAS FOR THE most part been associated with a process that's often done once or twice a year. It has been viewed much like spring cleaning where you get rid of things that have been sitting around the house all winter long. Unfortunately, this isn't what complete detoxification should be about. Spending two or three weeks trying to rid the body of toxins isn't going to have the long term benefits we all want to achieve. Your body is constantly exposed to toxins; there is a lot more that needs to be done to reduce overall body burden.

Remember, body burden is the total amount of toxic chemicals present in the body at any given time. As we've discussed, it's a kind of phantom number because we really can't calculate the total amount due to its varied distribution in the body. Toxins are not only found in the blood, they reside in tissues—especially in fat.

The conceptual calculation of body burden can be used as a baseline to understand how toxins can accumulate in the body.

> BODY BURDEN = Total Amount of Toxic Exposure –
> Body's Ability to Eliminate Toxins

Based on this equation we know that we need to reduce exposure and, at the same time, improve our body's own ability to get rid of toxins. In this chapter, our discussion will focus on how you can change your diet to enhance your body's ability to move toxins out. There are certain foods that can help you do this. Therefore, if you were to include these foods as part of your daily diet, then you would enhance detoxification pathways which, according to our equation, would lower overall body burden.

Also, since we consume so much food on a daily basis, reducing chemical exposure by making better food decisions will also reduce body burden. For example, choosing organic fruits and vegetables can reduce pesticide and chemical exposure. Note that over 80 percent of U.S. foods contain pesticides. By selecting certified organic foods, you minimize this exposure. Remember that the idea behind purchasing organic is not to improve nutrition but rather to reduce chemical exposure.

There are a number of easy adjustments you can make to your diet to improve detoxification mechanisms. Just by adding dietary fiber, you have already greatly improved your body's ability to get rid of toxins. Remember, fiber binds to toxins and gets them out of the body.

Eating ample amounts of protein, as well as lots of fruits and vegetables is also important to detoxification mechanisms. Protein supplies important amino acids for Phase II reactions, while fruits and vegetables not only support Phase II, they also supply antioxidants. In this chapter we are going to take an in-depth look at diet and the very important role it plays daily in helping you get rid of toxins.

DIETARY FIBER

Dietary fiber is perhaps one of the most important additions you can make to improve your overall health. As we've discussed in previous chapters, it's critical for binding toxin-laden bile and carrying it out of the body. Without the presence of fiber, bile gets re-absorbed back into the blood stream along with the chemical toxins it carries. A major change that has occurred in the Western diet is the reduction in the consumption of fiber, which has ultimately compromised detoxification.

Over 60 years ago, scientists began to study the effects of fiber on human health. At first, they believed that fiber had little to no nutritional value and was unimportant to the diet. During the grain milling process, bran (which is all fiber) was removed, leaving behind white, starchy flour stripped of fiber and other essential nutrients. This helped improve the functionality, appearance, and final flavor of the flour and bakers found it worked better for making bread and other baked products. But what they didn't realize was the detrimental effect this would have on health.

Research continued to evolve in this area, and scientists like Denis Burkitt, M.D., began looking at the differences in disease patterns between populations consuming a lot of refined foods versus those consuming little to no refined foods. Burkitt found that people on whole (unrefined) food diets typically did not experience constipation and other types of gastrointestinal disease like diverticulitis and Crohn's disease—diseases that are rampant in the Western population. It seemed that a steady diet of refined carbohydrates depleted the body of essential nutrients, leaving it unable to digest these carbohydrates. Although fiber does not have any nutritional value as it passes through the bowels undigested, it has many vital functions in the body. From this data, the research and medical communities began to understand the critical importance of fiber in the diet.

Scientific opinion has definitely evolved regarding fiber's role and we now know that a lack of this important nutrient also increases the body's toxic load. The National Cancer Institute has officially recognized fiber as an important element in the diet for the prevention of many cancers. As already discussed, a lack of dietary fiber can also lead to impaired digestion, bowel irregularities, diabetes, obesity, and heart disease. Yet, we still live in a fiber-deficient society. The majority of North Americans consume only one-quarter to one-half of the 2002 Institute of Medicine's recommended fiber levels of 38 grams per day for men and 25 grams per day for women. In fact, the average daily fiber intake is only 12 g for women and 18 g for men.

TYPES OF FIBER

As mentioned previously, there are two main types of fiber that are important for health: Soluble and insoluble. Soluble fiber refers to fiber material that can dissolve in water while insoluble refers to that fiber that cannot be dissolved in water. Soluble fiber is primarily found in oats, barley, and legumes, and in smaller amounts in fruits and vegetables. Soluble fiber forms a gel-like substance and works to increase the water content of the stools. Soluble fiber also acts as a binding agent to help soak up toxins, excess blood cholesterol, and sugar. It is also an important nutrient for the dietary management of high cholesterol and diabetes. A research study published in the *British Journal of Nutrition* confirmed these positive effects on persons consuming flaxseed daily. After four weeks, blood glucose levels were reduced by 27 percent while cholesterol levels were reduced by seven percent.

Research also shows that consuming sufficient amounts of insoluble fiber plays an important role in satiety (the feeling of fullness), and may help with weight management. Obesity is less prevalent in populations that consume a high-fiber diet.

Insoluble fiber is found in wheat, bran, and whole grains, and in smaller amounts in fruits and vegetables. It is not digested, even by bacteria in the gut, but it does give bulk to the stool. Insoluble fiber sweeps the colon, increases stool size, and helps relieve constipation and gas.

There are numerous benefits to consuming fiber. A high-fiber diet promotes increased chewing and slower eating, delays gastric emptying (which keeps you feeling fuller longer—up to four hours post-meal), stabilizes blood sugar levels, absorbs toxins, reduces cholesterol in the blood, increases stool size, makes stools softer ,and reduces your overall risk of chronic disease while maintaining a healthy digestive system.

FERMENTABLE FIBER

The American Association of Cereal Chemists defines soluble fiber this way: "The edible parts of plants or similar carbohydrates resistant to digestion and absorption in the human small intestine with complete or partial fermentation in the large intestine." Exactly what does that mean? Let's break it down:

EDIBLE PARTS OF PLANTS: Indicates that all parts of a plant we eat—skin, pulp, seeds, stems, leaves, and roots—contain fiber. Both insoluble and soluble sources are in those plant components.

CARBOHYDRATES: Complex carbohydrates, such as long-chained sugars (also called starch, oligosaccharides or polysaccharides), are excellent sources of fiber.

RESISTANT TO DIGESTION AND ABSORPTION IN THE HUMAN SMALL INTESTINE: Foods providing nutrients are digested by enzymes and acids in the stomach and small intestine where the nutrients are released then absorbed through the intestinal wall for transport via the blood throughout the body. A food resistant to this process is undigested, as insoluble and soluble fibers are. They pass to the large intestine only affected by their absorption of water (insoluble fiber) or dissolution in water (soluble fiber).

COMPLETE OR PARTIAL FERMENTATION IN THE LARGE INTESTINE: The large intestine comprises a segment called the colon within which additional nutrient absorption occurs through the process of fermentation. Fermentation occurs through the action of colonic bacteria on the food mass, producing gasses and short-chain fatty acids. It is these short-chain fatty acids—butyric, acetic, propionic, and valeric acids—that have such significant health properties.

SHORT-CHAIN FATTY ACIDS: Short-chain fatty acids are used by the intestinal mucosa or absorbed through the colonic wall into the portal circulation (supplying the liver) that transports them into the general circulatory system. Particularly, butyric acid has extensive physiological actions that promote health benefits.

Following is a list of the health benefits of butyric acid:

- Stabilizes blood glucose levels by acting on pancreatic insulin release (see diabetes chapter) and liver control of glycogen breakdown.
- Suppresses cholesterol synthesis by the liver and reduces blood levels of LDL cholesterol (bad cholesterol) and triglycerides responsible for atherosclerosis.

- Lowers colonic pH (i.e., raises the acidity level in the colon) which protects the lining from formation of colon polyps and increases the absorption of dietary minerals.
- Stimulates the production of T helper cells, antibodies, leukocytes, cytokines, and lymph mechanisms having crucial roles in immune protection.
- Increases the proliferation of colonic bacteria beneficial for intestinal health—*bifidobacteria* and *lactobacilli* (serving a probiotic function).
- Improves the barrier properties of the colonic mucosal layer, inhibiting inflammatory and adhesion irritants.

Summarizing these effects, fermentable fibers yield the important short-chain fatty acids that affect blood glucose and lipid levels, improves the colonic environment, and regulates immune responses. It's amazing to think that a compound like dietary fiber that never gets inside the blood stream can have so many indirect affects on human health.

START ROUGHING IT

Since dietary management is such an important part of improving digestive and bowel health, bringing your diet back to the "basics" is the best way to achieve an eating plan with adequate fiber content. Meat, dairy products, sugar, and fat contain no fiber. Processing removes the fiber from other foods. Consuming raw fruits and vegetables, whole grains, nuts, seeds, and legumes (peas, lentils and beans) is the best way to increase the fiber content of your diet and add phytonutrients rich in antioxidants.

Unfortunately, even though we are aware of the importance of these foods, we don't consume enough of them. We would rather grab fast foods that are high in fats and sugars. This creates many problems, including a compromised detoxification system.

FIBER IN FOODS

According to the Micronutrient Center of the Linus Pauling Institute, the five most fiber-rich plant foods are legumes (15-19 grams of fiber per one cup serving, including several types of beans, lentils, and peas), wheat bran (17 grams per cup), prunes (12 grams), Asian pear (10 grams each) and quinoa (9 grams).

Table 8.1 provides values for some foods that are good sources of fiber, reported as grams per 100 grams of edible portions, so that it is easy to compare foods. Information is given in the conversion column so that the value can be converted to the foods as normally eaten. Food preparation methods that remove or separate parts of the food also can alter fiber content. Raw oranges and orange juice have similar water content, but no fiber is present in the juice because the process of squeezing the fruit extracts the watery fraction and leaves behind the fiber associated with the pulp. The milling of whole grain removes fiber, which is concentrated in the outer bran layers of the cereal grain. White rice has lower fiber content than brown rice due to milling. A breakfast cereal made with wheat bran has a much higher fiber content than one made with a whole grain or a refined grain. When buying packaged food, take a look at the nutrition information to ensure you are purchasing the food with the highest fiber content. Also, begin looking at taking fiber as a daily supplement. I usually take my fiber before I go to bed at night in powder form. There are a number of good quality products on the market that provide natural, healthy fiber for proper detoxification. Fiber Fusion, PGX, and Viscofiber are products I often recommend.

FIBER SUPPLEMENTS

There are many types of soluble fiber supplements available for nutritional support. Many of these will help support detoxification mechanisms while others can help in the treatment of various gastrointestinal disorders. Others may help in lowering cholesterol and some may even reduce the risk of colon cancer. More recently there has been a renewed sense of excitement around fiber and its benefits in helping people reduce their weight. As we'll see in the next chapter, this association may also be related to fiber's ability to reduce chemical toxins in the body.

TABLE 9.1 Fiber content of some foods (source: Data obtained from the USDA Nutrient Database, release 13 at www.nal.usda.gov/fnic/foodcomp/)

Food Description	Dietary Fiber (g/100 g of edible portion)	Conversion Information
Fruits		
Bananas	2.4	1 medium = 118 g
Apples	2.7	1 medium = 138 g
Oranges	2.4	1 medium = 140 g
Orange juice	—	8 ounces = 248 g
Grapes	1.0	1 grape = 5 g
Plums, dried	7.1	1 dried plum = 8.4 g
Vegetables		
Tomatoes	1.1	1 medium = 123 g
Broccoli, cooked	2.9	1 spear = 37 g
Corn, cooked	2.4	½ cup = 82 g
Snap beans, cooked	2.8	1 cup = 124 g
Lettuce, romaine	1.7	½ cup = 28 g
Potatoes, baked without skin	1.5	½ cup = 61 g
Potatoes, French-fried, oven-baked	3.2	10 pieces
Peas, cooked	5.5	1 cup = 160 g
Cereals and Grains		
Bread, whole wheat	4.3	1 slice = 25 g
Bread, white	2.3	1 slice = 25 g
Bread, rye	5.8	1 slice = 32 g
Rice, white, cooked	0.4	1 cup = 158 g
Rice, brown, cooked	1.8	1 cup = 28 g
Oatmeal, cooked	2.3	
Bran Flakes	14.1	1 cup = 28 g
Corn Flakes	2.8	1 cup = 28 g
Dry Beans and Nuts		
Kidney beans, canned	3.5	
Garbanzo beans, canned	4.4	1 cup = 240 g
Almonds, dry-roasted	11.8	1 cup= 138 g
Walnuts, English	6.7	1 cup chopped = 120 g
Peanuts, dry-roasted	8.0	1 cup = 146 g

Fiber supplements come in capsules, tablets, powders, and sometimes even mixed in protein shakes. My preference has been powder form since I need to mix it with water. This assures me that I take enough water with the product. I always recommend a minimum of 8 ounces of water with 4 grams of fiber twice per day. Fiber Fusion comes in a number of great tasting flavors. Simply mix two teaspoons of the product with an 8 ounce glass of water in the morning and at night. You'll see improvement in overall bowel health in a very short period of time.

PSYLLIUM HUSK

Psyllium seed husk may reduce the risk of heart disease by lowering cholesterol levels. It also helps alleviate the symptoms of irritable bowel syndrome, although it often causes uncomfortable bloating. Psyllium husk is often labeled a "bulk-forming laxative," which can be misleading because it can also help diarrhea and it does not cause bowel dependency. The average amount of fiber consumed by Americans is 12 to 18 g daily while intake of 25 to 35 g per day is recommended by the FDA for a healthy diet. One way to achieve the recommended daily levels is with supplemental fiber like psyllium. Fiber Fusion contains a number of fiber ingredients including psyllium husks.

INULINS

Inulins are a group of oligosaccharides occurring naturally in many plants. They belong to a class of carbohydrates known as fructans. Inulin is used increasingly in prepared foods due to its favorable nutritional characteristics. Subtly sweet, it can be used to replace sugar, fat, and flour.

Inulin is advantageous because it contains 25 to 30 percent of the food energy of sugar or other carbohydrates and 10 to 15 percent of the food energy of fat. As a prebiotic fermentable fiber, it is metabolized by colonic bacteria yielding short-chain fatty acids. This increases the absorption of calcium and magnesium (among other potential beneficial effects) while promoting the health of intestinal bacteria. Inulin helps keep the GI environment in good working order, optimizing detoxification processes.

BETA-GLUCANS

Research into the soluble fiber components of dietary fiber has led to the discovery of fractions of oat soluble fiber, also called beta-glucans (found in the cell walls of grains). These fractions have been shown to effectively lower blood cholesterol, reduce postprandial blood glucose, induce satiety, suppress appetite, and even have immune stimulating properties.

Viscofiber is a superior natural ingredient with an enhanced concentration of soluble fiber (12 times more than oat bran). Viscofiber contains over 50 percent beta-glucans from oats and has an extremely high viscosity. The importance of viscosity has been accepted by the FDA and well documented by leading fiber scientists. It is the major property responsible for the physiological effects of consuming viscous soluble fiber such as lowering cholesterol and glucose levels. Fiber Fusion contains Viscofiber as a main ingredient.

VISCOUS FIBERS

Because soluble fiber disperses in water, a lot of soluble fiber is viscous (thick), allowing it to absorb and retain water as it forms a gel. Once a gel

TABLE 9.2 Soluble Fibers

Soluble Fiber	Source
Beta-glucan	Oats, barley
Inulin or fructo-oligosaccharide (FOS)	Chicory, Jerusalem artichokes, legumes (beans, lentils, dried peas)
Pectin	Apples, beets, orange peel, pears, strawberries, blueberries
Pentosans	Rye, wheat

TABLE 9.3 Insoluble Fiber

Insoluble Fibers	Sources
Agar	Seaweed
Cellulose	Grain and seed bran, couscous, barley, brown rice, bulgur
Lignin	Grain bran, flaxseed, pear

is formed, this type of soluble fiber actually slows down digestion, resulting in a feeling of fullness. This may contribute to weight control and has a tendency to stabilize blood sugar and permit better absorption of nutrients.

Another important attribute of viscous fiber is its ability to bind bile. Bile, as we have already mentioned, gets reabsorbed back into the circulation unless soluble fiber is present in the digestive tract. In the presence of viscous fiber, bile binds to it and gets excreted out of the body. The obvious benefit here is the fact that since toxins coming out of Phase II are attached to bile they also get excreted out of the body. A side effect of this bile excretion is lower cholesterol.

Viscous fibers have a grand role in the overall scheme of our health, especially detoxification. With that in mind, we should be doing everything we can to eat food that contributes viscous fiber.

FAT FACTS

So far we have focused on the benefits of fiber in overall health and in its ability to enhance detoxification mechanisms. Another nutritional element that has far reaching effects is fat. Having the right type of fat in your diet can enhance detoxification mechanisms while having the wrong fats can have the opposite outcome.

In the last fifteen years there has been much talk about reducing overall fat in the diet. A glimpse into the Western diet shows that increasing fat and sugar consumption, along with decreases in fiber, have contributed many of today's diseases. So although it seems reasonable to reduce the fat content in foods, we also need to understand that not all fats are created equal. There are certain fats that are essential for good health while others are detrimental to it.

Good fats are the unsaturated fats, namely the essential fatty acids. Then there are the bad fats that most of us eat daily. These fats get incorporated into our cells, which can lead to inflammation and a cell that is less responsive to external signals. In other words, when cell membranes (the outer core of cell) are made up of bad fats, the membrane becomes stiff, altering its physiological capabilities. The end result is it can slow down detoxification mechanisms.

SATURATED FATS: THE GOOD, THE NOT-SO-BAD, THE BAD, AND THE UGLY

Saturated fats are semisolid at room temperature and are found in animal products, such as red meat, pork, and lamb, and dairy products like milk, cheese, and butter. They are also included in many processed foods. They are generally considered "bad" fats because they can contribute to heart disease and obesity. Most health authorities recommend reducing saturated fats in the diet. However, not all saturated fats are created equally. There are three subgroups of saturated fats based on their chain length: short-chain, medium-chain, and long-chain fats.

Short-chain saturates, found in butter, coconut oil, and palm kernel oil, do not clog arteries, nor do they cause heart disease. Rather, they are easily digested and a source of fuel for energy.

Medium-chain saturates are found in several different foods, but the highest content is found in palm kernel and coconut oil. Medium-chain saturates are not associated with increasing cholesterol levels or the occurrence of heart disease. Medium-chain triglycerides (MCT oils) are used by athletes and dieters who want to convert fat into energy rather than store it as fat.

Long-chain saturates are the "bad" fats associated with raising LDL cholesterol, lowering HDL cholesterol, and increasing the risk of metabolic syndrome by causing insulin resistance and heart disease. The bad saturated fats are found in meat. Long-chain saturates are also a by-product of hydrogenation, a process that turns a liquid fat (at room temperature) into a solid and is employed in the manufacture of most margarines and shortening. Long-chain saturates are also abundant in restaurant fried foods, junk food, packaged baked goods, and processed foods. Hydrogenation or partial hydrogenation also distorts the fatty acids into a more poisonous form—trans fats.

Trans fat is by far the worst type of fat. Numerous research studies have shown that trans fats are more damaging to the heart than are saturated fats. The Institute of Medicine declared there is no safe level of trans fats and that consumption should be reduced as much as possible.

Trans fats were developed when there was a backlash against saturated fats. They are artificial, formed by a process of high temperature and hydrogenation that turns refined oils into margarines, shortenings, and partially hydrogenated vegetable oils, making them solid or semi-solid and "shelf stable. Our bodies cannot recognize them as nutrients and therefore are not able to process them. They are, however, a food manufacturer's dream as they are inexpensive to produce and extend the shelf life of foods.

These man-made fats are found everywhere in your cupboard, yet I would bet many people don't even know they are eating them. Trans fats have been dubbed "phantom fats" because, until recently, the labeling of trans fats was not mandatory. Thankfully, now you can pick up a box of crackers and see what the trans fat content is, then make the right decision for your heart and waistline—and put the crackers back on the shelf if they contain trans fats.

Table 9.4 contains a list of the trans fats found in some common foods.

What do these bad and ugly fats have to do with detoxification? Besides causing the problems we've just discussed, bad and ugly fats can impact detoxification mechanisms. They can become incorporated

TABLE 9.4 Trans Fat Content of Some Common Foods

Vegetable Shortening	1.4 – 4.2
Margarine (stick)	1.8 – 3.5
Margarine (tub, regular)	0.4 – 1.6
Salad Dressings (regular)	0.06 – 1.1
Vegetable Oils	0.01 – 0.06
Pound cake	4.3
Doughnuts	0.3 – 3.8
Microwave Popcorn	2.2
Chocolate Chip Cookies	1.2 – 2.7
French Fries (fast food)	0.7 – 3.6
Snack Crackers	1.8 – 2.5

into various tissues (cell membranes specifically) that are important to detoxification mechanisms—the liver cells, gastrointestinal cells, skin cells, and so on. These fats can alter how efficiently these cells function.

As we discussed in earlier chapters, the cell membrane is the outer shell of the cell. When cell membranes are healthy, they are flexible and permeable so that nutrients can travel into the cell and waste can travel out. But saturated and trans fats can damage cell membranes so that they don't function optimally—and this can impede detoxification. In other words, the waste cannot be eliminated from the cells.

OMEGA-3'S TO THE RESCUE

For many years, I have recommended that my patients include high quality omega-3 fish oils in their diet. I am sure you have heard about the benefits of fish oil for heart health, diabetes, depression, and even brain development. The literature on fish oil is significant. Original observations were seen in the people of Greenland and the Inuits who had low rates of cardiovascular disease. Researchers linked these low levels of heart disease to the consumption of cold water fish containing high levels of omega-3 fatty acids, specifically EPA and DHA.

Follow-up studies have indeed proven that these specific omega-3 fatty acids not only have cardio-protective properties but other benefits that are now being researched. When it comes to detoxification, EPA and DHA have the ability to be incorporated into cellular membranes thus improving cell function.

FRUITS, VEGETABLES, AND DETOXIFICATION

We have talked about two important nutrients in your detoxification daily diet regime. I keep emphasizing daily, because even though we want to carry out detoxification treatments at least three times per year, we also want to support detoxification mechanisms throughout the year. This means learning about what important dietary changes and/or additions need to be made to achieve such affects.

Thus far, we've talked about one of the most important components you can add to your diet—dietary fiber. We've also discussed the importance of essential fats and the major contribution they can make to general health. But it's also important to include lots of fresh fruits and vegetables in your diet.

Today, virtually every government agency recommends eating fruits and vegetables—eight servings a day. Studies show that fruits and vegetables can protect us from all sorts of ailments, including cancer. The protective properties in these foods have not only been linked to their vitamin and mineral content, but also the very precious substances known as phytochemicals.

Increasing your daily consumption of fruits and vegetables not only improves your overall general health, it can greatly assist your detoxification pathways in two different ways. First, it can supply the important antioxidants needed to quench the high levels of free radicals produced during Phase I detoxification. Second, specific types of vegetables can help support detoxification pathways by enhancing chemical reactions.

ANTIOXIDANT EFFECTS

As we learned earlier, antioxidants are important in reducing the harmful effects of toxins and controlling the damaging effects of Phase I intermediates. The body has its own powerful antioxidant known as glutathione. But because of the unnaturally high toxic load constantly coming into the body, glutathione levels can be compromised. An important step in supporting this aspect of detoxification is to supplement with antioxidants.

A natural method of doing this is by making sure you are eating ample amounts of fresh fruits and vegetables. Both fruits and vegetables have naturally occurring antioxidants that not only act as direct antioxidants but can also support the production of glutathione. These include vitamin C (ascorbic acid), carotenes like lycopene and lutein, polyphenols, and dozens of other phytochemicals. Many of these ingredients directly quench free radicals while others, like vitamin C, help in the regeneration and production of glutathione. To get the benefit from these antioxidants, make sure to eat plenty of highly colored fruits and vegetables every day.

IMPORTANT DETOXIFICATION FOODS

Did you know that a variety of fruits and vegetables have nutrients that actually support detoxification mechanisms? Some can support detoxification enzymes in the liver while others can enhance bile movement both in the liver and gallbladder. Simply adding some of these foods to your daily diet can help reduce your overall body burden.

CRUCIFEROUS VEGETABLES: Cruciferous vegetables belong to the family of edible plants known as brassicaceae. These include broccoli, Brussels sprouts, cauliflower, cabbage, collard greens, and rapini. These vegetables contain a number of important nutrients, making them extremely beneficial for general health. They are high in vitamin C and soluble fiber but, more impressively, they contain multiple nutrients with well-known anti-cancer properties. These include diindolylmethane, sulforaphane, and selenium.

Due to these compounds, cruciferous vegetables can stimulate both Phase I and Phase II detoxification pathways as well being powerful antioxidants. Making cruciferous vegetables a part of your daily diet not only aids in helping detoxification mechanisms, it also helps provide antioxidant support.

Recommendation: One-half cup per day.

SULFUR VEGETABLES: Onions and garlic are rich in a variety of organic sulfur compounds. Studies show both of these vegetables help lower blood pressure and cholesterol levels, regulate blood sugar and provide antibiotic effects. These foods also have the ability to help with one of the Phase II conjugation pathways known as sulfation. Food additives, certain drugs, and intestinal bacterial toxins are neutralized by sulfation reactions.

Recommendations: One clove of garlic per day and handful of cooked onions.

CITRUS FRUITS: Lemons, oranges, and limes have had a long history of use and have been considered beneficial by the majority of the population. These fruits are high in vitamin C phytochemicals that have powerful antioxidant effects. These compounds can quench free radicals and thus support the body's detoxification pathways. Recent studies have also centered on limonene, a phytochemical found in citrus that may have gallstone dissolving properties and possible anticancer activity. But limonene also seems to enhance Phase II activity specifically glutathione conjugation and glucoronidation reactions.

Recommendations: One orange per day and half a lemon squeezed into 8 ounces of water.

POMEGRANATE, RASPBERRIES, AND STRAWBERRIES: These fruits contain ellagic acid, a phenolic compound that has some excellent detoxification properties. Ellagic acid not only acts as an antioxidant but also has liver protective effects and can support Phase II detoxification enzymes. Some research is also pointing in the direction that ellagic acid may help in the prevention of cancer.

Recommendations: A great way to get ellagic acid in your diet is to drink pomegranate juice (I recommend 3 oz daily of POM Wonderful).

BILE MOVERS: Bile is produced in the liver and stored in the gallbladder. One of the important functions of bile is to move toxins from the liver to the gallbladder and eventually into the duodenum. Artichokes, dandelions, and beets have all been shown to help move bile more efficiently. Artichokes contain cynarin which not only improves the flow of bile in the liver but also helps lower cholesterol. Dandelion has a long history of use in liver conditions and has been shown to enhance the movement of bile from both the liver and the gallbladder. Animal studies have also shown dandelion to significantly increase the clearance of toxins. Beets also improve detoxification processes.

Recommendations: Include one-half cup (combined) of these foods as mixtures in salads.

DETOXIFICATION WITH FOOD

Changing lifestyles and eating habits are key factors in improving overall well-being. Yet very few people regard lifestyle and food as essential elements in optimizing detoxification mechanisms. Altering the diet by adding high fiber foods, cruciferous vegetables, onions and garlic, beets and dandelion, and citrus fruits can go a long way in helping you reduce overall body burden.

10

CHAPTER TEN

Epigenetics And Detoxification

IN 2003, ONE OF HUMANKIND'S GREATEST intellectual achievements was realized. That was the year that the human genome, through a multinational effort, had been mapped. The genome is the full set of genetic instructions for a living thing, controlling its development from a single cell into a complex adult body. This discovery opened the door to a whole new set of possibilities that could answer many of the mysteries of human disease.

The Human Genome Project identified an estimated 30,000 to 35,000 genes carried by the 23 pairs of chromosomes (46 in total) found in nearly every cell of the body. This gave us our first look into the very thing that makes us who we are. Never in human history had we come so close to the blueprint of creation itself, peeking into the mysteries of human existence.

This project not only identified the genes, it also found that only three percent of these genes carry actual data to make things like proteins and other substances. The rest of the information carried in genes is called non-coding and junk DNA (meaning that it doesn't seem to have any purpose). But as we all know, Mother Nature has a function for everything, so the rest of the 97 percent of the information found in the genes may have purposes we have yet to uncover.

The goal of this chapter is to help you gain an understanding about the human genome, its chromosomes, it genes, and ultimately its DNA. Understanding how it all works is critical to forming an appreciation as to why it is so important for us to reduce chemical exposure and improve our body's ability to get rid of chemical toxins. It is ultimately here, within the genes, that chemicals cause the damage creating the health problems we are desperately trying to avoid.

WHAT IS THE HUMAN GENOME?

The Human Genome is the 23 pairs of chromosomes found in every single cell of your body. This is the instruction manual on how to make "you," carrying within it information on height and the color of your eyes, hair and skin. It also carries information on how intelligent you will become and how well you will age. Structurally, each chromosome consists of hundreds of genes which are made up of DNA.

When we think about the fact that almost every single cell in your body carries all 23 pairs of chromosomes a question comes to mind; how do cells in your heart know that they should make proteins to make your heart beat instead of making proteins for hearing? The answer to this question is important to understand—not only how genes work but also how the environment can alter the way genes are read.

All the information necessary for a living being to grow and live is found inside the nucleus of every cell. These instructions tell a cell what role it will play in your body. The environment of the nucleus will inform that cell which of the 30,000 genes should be turned on and which ones should remain off. This is an intricate task only achieved through the incredible intelligence of the genes sensing their environment.

DNA

The instructions come in the form of a molecule called deoxyribonucleic acid (DNA). DNA encodes a detailed set of plans, a blueprint for building part of a cell. Its structure is the famous double helix (Figure 10.1), a twisted ladder whose steps are built with the

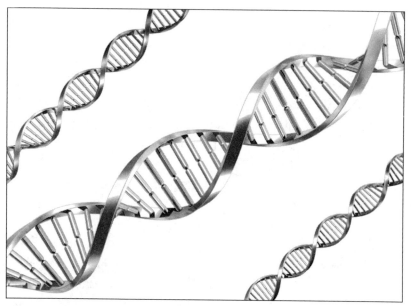

FIGURE 10.1 The double helix DNA molecule

four letter DNA alphabet. The alphabet pieces, A, C, T and G come together in a specific arrangement; A always binds with C and T always joins with G.

The DNA strand is made up of these letters which make up the words in your instruction manual, which become sections in chapters. These sections are the genes and the chapters are the chromosomes. It is the genes that tell the cell to make molecules (proteins). Proteins enable a cell to perform special functions, such as working with other groups of cells to make the heart beat, etc.

GENES

Genes are the specific directions for building all the proteins that make our bodies function. DNA is made up of genes. For example, one long strand of DNA may contain many genes. All together there are over 30,000 genes. If you consider eye color, there are just a few of these genes that produce proteins that code for the color. This creates an enzyme that produces a pigment to give you your eye color. But if something causes damage to these genes or changes the way the body reads them, then you may have a mutation (change in the genes) and get a completely different eye color.

CHROMOSOMES

DNA is packaged into compact units called chromosomes. To do this, the double helix wraps around some proteins which are then packed tightly together until they from a chromosome. There are 23 pairs of chromosomes in each cell (for a total of 46); one comes from the mother and the other from the father.

SIMPLIFYING IT

To make this whole idea of the genome, chromosomes, genes and DNA a bit easier to understand, lets look once again at a simplified analogy—a manual. The genome is the instruction manual on how to make

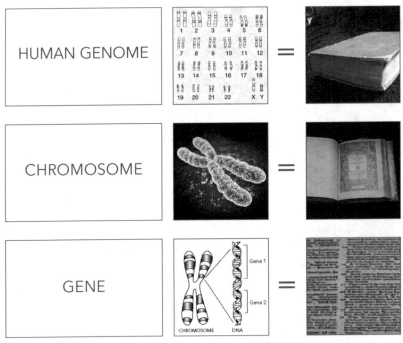

FIGURE 10.2 DNA, the human manual on how to make you

you, the 23 chromosomes are the 23 chapters in that manual. Within those chapters are sections and those sections are the genes. The words in the sections are your DNA. A little simplistic, but you get the picture (Fig 10.2).

Genetics has evolved rapidly since the genome project was completed in 2003. We are constantly learning more about genes and their relationship with health and disease. The ongoing research is giving us new clues on how to predict whether or not individuals are at risk for diseases and possibly, one day, how we can alter their course.

But there really is nothing more exciting, nothing that offers more hope and insight, than the new science of genetics known as epigenetics.

EPIGENETICS DEFINED

Epigenetics refers to changes that occur in gene expression caused by factors other than the DNA itself. As we have just learned, the genome is basically the instruction manual on making the human body. Taking this one step further, we have to conclude that genes themselves also need instruction for what to do, and where and when to do it. For example, a human heart cell contains the exact same DNA as a liver cell, yet that heart cell knows to code only for those proteins needed for heart function. How the heart cell knows which genes it needs to turn on lies not in the DNA but on it, in the form of switches that can turn genes on and off. This whole switch system is known as the epigenome; the field is called epigenetics.

The interesting aspect about this is that there is no change in the underlying DNA sequence, instead, non-genetic factors cause the organism's genes to behave differently. These non-genetic factors could be certain vitamins, minerals, toxins or even emotions that can turn on or off specific genes, impacting the way they express themselves. Even more surprising is that epigenetic signals can be passed from one generation to the next.

In the last decade there has been a growing body of evidence supporting the impact that epigenetics has on who we become. The

Discover article we discussed earlier focused on the new science of epigenetics and how it is rewriting the rules of not only disease, but heredity and identity.

One of the studies it reviews is a breakthrough experiment conducted by Randy Jirtile, Ph.D., professor of radiation oncology at Duke University. Dr. Jirtile and his colleagues started with a group of agouti mice. These mice carry the agouti gene that makes them fat, yellow, and prone to diabetes and cancer. When agouti mice breed, the offspring are identical to the parents—fat, yellow and prone to disease. The goal of the experiment was to see if they could change the fate of these mice by changing the mother's diet. The results of the experiment were nothing short of astounding.

In the experimental group given the new diet, the offspring looked nothing like their parents. They were slender, brown in color, and did not display a propensity for cancer and diabetes that their parents were susceptible to. In fact these mice lived to a ripe old age. The end result was that the effects of the agouti gene had suddenly vanished.

So, what happened? Before conception, the researchers began feeding the test group of mother mice with a special diet rich in methyl donors (small molecule that can attach themselves to a gene and turn it off). These molecules are common in the environment and found in many foods including garlic, onions and folic acid supplements often given to pregnant women. Once this diet was given to the agouti mice mothers, these methyl donors worked their way into the embryo's chromosomes and eventually into the agouti gene. The mothers passed the agouti gene to the offspring, but because of the methyl rich diet, the chemical switch turned off the gene's effects. The end result was that the agouti gene was not altered at all; it was exactly the same gene that had been passed on from generation to generation. But what did change was the epigenome—the switch that controls the expression of the gene.

In my years as a physician, I believe this was one of the great insights into how important the environment actually is. To think that we can make such dramatic impacts on the gene expression of a baby just by changing the mother's diet is unbelievable. How many babies worldwide are being effected by the environment? How many of these babies are developing all sorts of new diseases through this same mechanism?

Even though we can't fully answer these questions, it gives us insight into the fact that environmental pollution and the hundreds of chemical toxins are having a negative impact and possibly contributing to many of the health issues we face today.

ENVIRONMENT CAN IMPACT GENETICS

What if I were to tell you that the food you eat, the water you drink, the things your skin comes in contact with, and the love and attention you get at home can have a big impact on not only your inner physiology, but the way you look? It is a definite change from thinking that we inherit all of our traits and weaknesses. When patients come into my office for the first time, they fill out a medical history form that contains a section that asks about family history of illnesses. Yet now, through scientific research and a better understanding of epigenetics, we have suddenly learned a whole new set of rules. We have learned that, just because your parents have heart disease or cancer, doesn't mean you are going to have the same problems. The main reason why you develop the same diseases is because you do exactly the same things your parents did. In other words, if you eat the same food, live in the same area, and work in the same environment, chances are the same types of triggers will impact your genetics as well.

As I mentioned earlier, Hippocratic physicians talked about this very thing nearly 2,500 years ago. Their philosophy was that we should look for disease in the environment, in the food we eat, in the water we drink, and in the air we breathe. Nearly 2,500 years later, science has validated their concepts in ways that touch the core of human existence.

How many of us have suspected that environmental factors not only have an impact on the health of our planet but also on every living creature? Many of us have thought about it, but not truly believed it. All of that is now changing; epigenetics is the root of this change and ultimately could be at the foundation of what solves our health problems.

Epigenetics is one of the most eye opening and exciting fields of medicine. To think that we can change the behavior of our genes by improving our environment! As a physician, it is sometimes difficult to grasp and other times nothing short of miraculous.

In many ways it validates that idea of a pure environment. It validates the concept of good nutrition. And it validates the concept that healthy living—physically, nutritionally, and spiritually. All of these factors play critical roles in what we become. Based on our knowledge of epigenetics, detoxifying could pay huge dividends.

With the knowledge we have about epigenetics, we can understand the importance of detoxification. The notion that measuring body burden can reveal anywhere from 400 to 700 chemicals in our bodies at any given time is disturbing. What effect is this having on gene behavior? The effects are obvious as we've seen in both animal and human observational studies. Very few will argue about the link between cancer and the environment such as toxic chemicals like pesticides. However, in order for this information to be truly meaningful, we must leverage this knowledge to change our views of the effects of toxic chemicals and ultimately our views of the environment. We must also use this information to accomplish successful detoxification.

CHAPTER ELEVEN

Weight Loss: A New View

IT'S NO SECRET THAT OBESITY IS the nation's leading health problem. The number of individuals who are obese has continued to escalate to the point of being labeled an epidemic by the U.S. government. Every year, more and more people become overweight, eventually becoming obese. Today, more than 30 percent of Americans are clinically obese and, since 1985, the number of overweight children has doubled. If left untreated, obesity poses a serious threat to future generations. According to William J. Klish, M.D., professor of pediatrics at the Baylor College of Medicine, "Children today have a shorter life expectancy than their parents for the first time in 100 years." This should be a concern to every citizen. When our greatest resource—our children—have a shorter life expectancy than their parents, we should all be troubled. We need to become versed in the contributing factors to this problem and then acquire the necessary tools to turn it around. Learning about toxic chemicals and their effects on the human body may turn out to be an important factor necessary in overcoming the hurdles that have, for decades, blocked people from achieving their optimal body weight.

In this chapter, we'll look at why obesity has become an epidemic. Even with the hundreds of new diet books that come out each year, the pounds just keep accumulating.

WHAT'S SO BAD ABOUT BEING OVERWEIGHT?

It's no secret that overweight and obese individuals have more health issues than people with ideal body weight. Medical science tells us that these individuals have more heart disease, diabetes, high blood pressure, and cancer—and they are more prone to an early death. Many obese and overweight individuals know these facts and are constantly trying to find the magic bullet to change their circumstances.

Visualizing what excess weight can do sometimes helps give the motivation needed for change. For example, I usually tell my patients to visualize carrying a 20 pound bag of potatoes on their backs for a few days. I then ask them how they would feel. Their responses are uncannily similar; they say they would probably have a sore back, that they would definitely feel tired, and that they probably couldn't do the things they normally did. Yet, this is exactly how an overweight person feels! But being overweight or obese doesn't just trigger these physical symptoms. There are social and behavioral consequences as well.

So why don't people just lose the weight? People in America genuinely want to be healthy, but they consistently fail because the things they do to lose weight just don't seem to work long term. You begin a diet, it works for a month, maybe two, and then things just begin to fall apart again. It's a constant struggle, an uphill battle that seems to take more work than anybody is willing to do. In the end, most people give up and go back to their old habits. As a result, they gain their weight back and, in some cases, even more.

One of the frustrating things about trying to lose weight is seeing a friend who eats twice as much as you yet never seems to put on a pound. Why does somebody who eats whatever they want not gain weight? Most of us have always assumed that these people have fast metabolisms. This makes sense. But why do they have a faster metabolism? Is it genetic or is there something else at work? Let's take a closer look.

OUR GROWING WAISTLINES

Obesity is the most common nutritional disorder in the industrialized world today. There are ominous statistics everywhere we turn:

- The percentage of children and adolescents who are obese has doubled in the past 20 years.
- Researchers estimate that obesity causes about 300,000 deaths in the United States annually.
- Obesity is fueling the rise in Type II diabetes, which also reduces lifespan.
- The prevalence of obesity in U.S. adults has increased about fifty percent per decade since 1980.
- According to the *New England Journal of Medicine*, studies suggest that two-thirds of American adults are overweight—they have a body mass index (BMI) of 25 or more—or obese—indicated by a BMI of 30 or more.
- Thirty percent of adults age 20 and older are obese.
- Fifteen percent of children age six to 11 and 30 percent age 12 to 19 are obese.
- Obesity costs $117 billion a year.

According to the World Health Organization (WHO), the best way to determine an overweight or obese adult is by using something called the body mass index (BMI). This uses weight in kilograms divided by the square of height in meters, or weight in pounds multiplied by 705, then divided twice by height in inches. A BMI between 25 and 29.9 indicates that an individual is overweight; an obese adult has a BMI of 30 or higher. The higher your BMI, the greater your risk of developing health problems. (see table 6.1).

One variable the BMI fails to consider is lean body mass (tissue, bone, and muscle), which weighs significantly more than fat does. It is possible for a healthy, muscular individual to be classified as obese using the BMI formula. If you are a trained athlete, your weight—based on a measured percentage of body fat—would be a better indicator of what you should weigh. The average healthy man should not exceed 15 percent body fat, while the healthy limit for a woman is 15 to 22 percent.

TABLE 11.1   BMI CALCULATIONS

BMI (kg/m²)	19	20	21	22	23	24	25	26	27	28	29	30	35	40
Height (in.)	Weight (lb.)													
58	91	96	100	105	110	115	119	124	129	134	138	143	167	191
59	94	99	104	109	114	119	124	128	133	138	143	148	173	198
60	97	102	107	112	118	123	128	133	138	143	148	153	179	204
61	100	106	111	116	122	127	132	137	143	148	153	158	185	211
62	104	109	115	120	126	131	136	142	147	153	158	164	191	218
63	107	113	118	124	130	135	141	146	152	158	163	169	197	225
64	110	116	122	128	134	140	145	151	157	163	169	174	204	232
65	114	120	126	132	138	144	150	156	162	168	174	180	210	240
66	118	124	130	136	142	148	155	161	167	173	179	186	216	247
67	121	127	134	140	146	153	159	166	172	178	185	191	223	255
68	125	131	138	144	151	158	164	171	177	184	190	197	230	262
69	128	135	142	149	155	162	169	176	182	189	196	203	236	270
70	132	139	146	153	160	167	174	181	188	195	202	207	243	278
71	136	143	150	157	165	172	179	186	193	200	208	215	250	286
72	140	147	154	162	169	177	184	191	199	206	213	221	258	294
73	144	151	159	166	174	182	189	197	204	212	219	227	265	302
74	148	155	163	171	179	186	194	202	210	218	225	233	272	311
75	152	160	168	176	184	192	200	208	216	224	232	240	279	319
76	156	164	172	180	189	197	205	213	221	230	238	246	287	328

CALCULATING BMI

To calculate your BMI, check table 6.2. Find your height in inches along the left column. Then follow that row to your current weight. The number at the top of that height-weight intersection is your BMI. If your BMI is 24 or less, congratulations, you are within a healthy weight. However if you are above 25 then follow the graph back and find your ideal weight for height at a BMI of 24. This will give you a goal to work toward.

TABLE 11.2 Body Weight Classifications in Adults

Body Mass Index	Classification	Descriptor
<18.5	Underweight	May be associated with health problems for some people
18.5 to 24.9	Normal weight	Good weight for most people
25.0 to 29.9	Overweight	Increasing risk of developing health problems
>30	Obese	High risk of developing health problems

Source: World Health Organization, Obesity: Preventing and Managing the Global Epidemic, WHO technical report series no. 894 (Geneva: World Health Organization, 2000); Health Canada, Canadian Guidelines for Body Weight Classification in Adults (Ottawa: Health Canada 2003).

Many of you will be happy to hear that you might be able to throw your scale away! Weight lose experts are moving away from the scale in accordance with the National Cholesterol Education's recommendations for determining overweight and obese individuals. Instead of the scale, we are going to use the tape measure as a way of determining where and how your body fat is distributed. Your waist-to-hip ratio can be calculated by dividing your waist measurement (at the narrowest point; women should aim for a waist under 32.5 inches and men under 35 inches) by your hip measurement (at the widest point). Women with waist-to-hip ratios of more than 0.8 and men with waist-to-hip ratios of more than 1.0 are at an increased health risk because of their fat distribution. It is healthier to be "pear" shaped with more fat stored below the waistline than it is to be "apple" shaped with fat stored around the abdominal section. People who store fat around their waistline have an increased risk of Type II diabetes and cardiovascular disease.

Eating more calories than we burn in a day causes the caloric balance to accumulate. It's a concept that's easy to understand, but not one that's necessarily easy to practice—even though more of us have become aware of the consequences to our health and our looks.

Data from the United States and Canada shows us that food consumption is increasing. There have been overall increases in soft drink and sugar consumption. It is estimated that the average American consumes about 150 pounds of refined sugar and 60 pounds of high fructose corn syrup per year, much of it from the things we drink. In surveys of middle school children, this sweetened soft drink consumption was associated with increased BMI and obesity.

RESTAURANTS AND FAST FOOD

The increase in eating food away from home—particularly in fast-food restaurants—is not surprising considering that, in the United States, the number of fast-food restaurants grew 147 percent from 1972 to 1995, and the percentage of meals and snacks consumed at fast-food restaurants doubled. Eating at a fast-food restaurant is associated with increased calorie and fat intake, largely due to increases in high-fat, high-sugar food choices such as French fries and soft drinks, and decreases in the consumption of fruits, vegetables, and milk. Even our grocery stores have changed to reflect our fast food mentality. The change from small neighborhood grocery stores to large supermarkets has been positively associated with increased caloric intake. Why?. Because supermarkets offer a greater variety of processed and convenience foods. What do fast food restaurants and the processed foods we buy at the supermarket have in common? They all contain added chemicals to preserve the food, enhance its flavor, and make it look better. In other words, all of these foods have toxic chemicals that may have a detrimental effect on human physiology.

An increase in the amount of calories we consume can also be partly blamed on larger portion sizes. Examinations of trends in food portion sizes in the United States from 1977 to 1998 found that portion sizes and energy intake increased for all key foods (except pizza) at all locations, with the largest portions consumed at fast-food restaurants. "Super sizing" of portions is one of the greatest contributors. For example, the current McDonald's "child-size" soft drink is twelve ounces; the same serving size in the 1950s would have been marketed as "king-size." A study comparing the USDA's recommended serving size and what is currently being sold in the marketplace reveals that serving sizes now exceed the standards: soda by 35 percent; fast-food hamburgers by 112 percent; bagels by 195 percent; steak by 224 percent; and cookies by 700 percent. Portion sizes began to grow in the 1970s, although fewer than ten large-sized portions were introduced in that decade. The number of larger sizes rose sharply in the 1980s and has continued to increase steadily. Between 1995 and 1999, sixty-five new large-size portions were introduced.

Exposure to food advertising may also influence the purchase of foods with more calories, more chemicals, and less nutritional value. Foods that are heavily advertised are generally over-consumed relative to recommendations, while foods that are advertised less frequently are under consumed. We don't see many television commercials for organic fruits and vegetables, but there are numerous ones for fast-food restaurants and soft drinks. In 1997 (the most recent reported), U.S. food manufacturers and retailers spent $11 billion in mass-marketing media advertising. This amount included $765 million on confectioneries and snacks, $571 million on McDonald's, $549 million on soft drinks, and $105 million on fruits and vegetables. The entire nutrition education budget for the USDA that same year was $333 million (or three percent of food industry expenditures). These food advertisements generally reflect the types of foods being consumed. And it's these foods that are to blame for an increased risk of obesity, tooth decay, cardiovascular disease, and Type II diabetes.

FAD DIETS

Atkins, Beverly Hills, Cabbage Soup, Apple Cider Vinegar, Eat Right 4 Your Blood Type, Grapefruit, Ornish, South Beach, Sugar Busters, Zone—the list of weight loss diets goes on and on. I'm sure most of you have heard of them and some of you may have even tried a few. Did you ever wonder why there are so many fad diets out there? It's because people are looking for that quick fix to help them lose those extra pounds that are hanging around the waist, hips, and thighs. But the sad truth is that fad diets don't work, at least not on a long term basis. They are a multibillion dollar industry that offers a variety of products, all with magical claims. In many cases, once you go off the diet, not only do you regain the weight lost but you'll probably add some extra weight as well. The diet industry's success is built on our failures.

Why don't these fad diets help you lose weight or keep the weight off? Fad diets are generally so unrealistic and so unpleasant that they cannot be maintained for the long term. Most of us trying to lose weight will stop the diet because it's too restrictive in food choices, too boring, too expensive, and too stressful. Plus, a 2004 study published in the *Annals of Internal Medicine* demonstrated that there is little evidence to support the use of many of these commercial weight-loss programs.

A study published in the *Journal of the American Dietetic Association* in September 2005 confirmed that women who want to lose weight should place emphasis on dietary fiber rather than on low-carb, low-fat, and high-protein diets. The study was based on the 4,539 people who participated in the Continuing Survey of Food Intakes between 1994 and 1996. The survey found that only five percent reported an adequate intake of fiber. It also found that, for women, a low-fiber, high-fat diet increased the risk of being overweight or obese. Beyond weight control, the researchers noted that a fiber-rich diet provides a wide range of health benefits for both men and women, such as lower blood cholesterol levels, a reduced risk of digestive diseases, and a possible reduction in the risk of heart disease. In light of these benefits, the researchers concluded that increased fiber consumption should be promoted to both men and women.

But what the researchers didn't talk about is the fact that fiber is an important component in detoxification. As we've learned, fiber is the component that binds bile, the ingredient that is carrying chemical toxins and excretes out of the body. Another thing the researchers missed is the link between environmental pollution and obesity.

A NEW PARADIGM

An area of obesity that hasn't been fully explored or often discussed is the impact of environmental toxins and weight gain. The obesity epidemic just gets worse, even though we have dozens of new diets, hundreds of new diet books, thousands of low calorie foods, and billions and billions of dollars spent every year on this condition.

A plausible explanation for this might lie in the vast number of chemical toxins we are exposed to. Research is beginning to show that environmental chemicals can have an impact on the weight control centers in the body. Both animal and human models suggest that various aspects of the endocrine system and sympathetic nervous system can be affected by chemical toxins, which may then disrupt important hormonal weight control systems within the body. This could possibly explain why people continually gain weight and why a greater percentage of the North American population is becoming obese. Even though there are more fitness centers than ever before, even though more people are exercising and making better food choices, the statistics keep getting worse. Something is up and chemical toxins could be a major factor in this epidemic.

A STUDY CAUGHT MY EYE

Reviewing literature is something that physicians do on a regular basis in order to keep up with the ever-changing landscape of medicine. I usually look for research validating the nutritional aspects of health care, such as the scientific validation of plant ingredients, vitamins, minerals, and amino acids. In 2002, I came across an article in the *Journal of Toxicology* titled "Weight Loss and The Release of Toxic Chemicals." The study followed a group of people on a weight loss program that included calorie restriction and in some cases weight loss medication. Various parameters were measured that included, fat loss, weight loss, blood levels of chemical toxins, T3 and T4 thyroid hormone counts and RMR(Resting Metabolic Rate). My interest centered on the toxic chemical levels and the T3 (active thyroid hormone).

As I mentioned previously, it's a well-established fact that chemical toxins, including pesticides, are stored in our fat tissues. This is significant because this is one of the ways the body gets rid of these chemicals when the liver can't keep up and there is a high level of them in the blood stream. But when people use saunas or go on fasts or weight loss programs that break down body fat, the bound chemical toxins are released. In this particular study, DDT, DDE, and PCBs were measured. The levels of all three toxins rose significantly as the patients began losing weight. But what is really fascinating about this study was that the T3 count dropped in all the participants. T3 is also known as active thyroid hormone. It is the messenger that speeds up your metabolism. When people have low levels of T3, they tend to gain weight easily, they feel cold in their extremities and they are very tired. These people are usually diagnosed with low thyroid and are usually placed on levothyroxine, a synthetic thyroid medication that increases T3.

In this particular study, as subjects lost weight, the levels of toxic chemicals in their blood rose which, in turn had an impact on the production of T3. The end result was a reduction in thyroid hormone which created a sudden drop in RMR. This reduced metabolic rate makes losing weight even more difficult. It also makes gaining weight a lot easier.

This opens up a whole new world of possibilities for weight loss programs. If these toxic chemicals affect the thyroid, what other metabolic systems that control weight gain are they affecting? And if so, could this be the reason why so many people gain weight?

CONSIDER THIS

I've noticed some interesting observations in my clinical practice— things you may have also seen in your friends, co-workers, and family members.

- The person who eats large amounts of food and doesn't exercise but never gains weight. How many of us have been frustrated by this type of individual? We assume that this type of person just naturally has a high metabolism or good genes. But DNA doesn't necessarily dictate what you become. What if this type of person had an ability to clear toxins that attach to his/her weight control centers better than most of the population? What if this person wasn't affected by chemicals that might affect others?

  Scientifically, this is plausible because we know that polymorphisms exist in the detoxification pathways. This is why some people can easily clear caffeine and others can't. If this individual had this capacity, it would explain why he or she maintained their weight. This validates the chemical toxin theory.

- On the opposite end of the spectrum, there is the person who doesn't eat much but is obese anyway. We have all seen this type of person. The fact that they remain overweight even though they don't consume large amounts of calories seems perplexing. But what is really happening is that their weight control mechanisms just aren't working properly. This, again, may be related to chemical exposure.

- There has been a lot of research on the benefits of fiber and weight loss. We know with great certainty that fiber not only controls blood sugar levels but it also gives us a feeling of fullness which can help in weight loss program. We also know that fiber— specifically soluble fiber—binds the bile that carries toxins from the liver to the GI tract for excretion. Research shows that, only in the presence of fiber, can bile be excreted out of the body. If fiber is not present, nearly 98 percent of this toxin-filled bile is absorbed back into the body. So, along with fiber's ability to promote a feeling of fullness, it may also aid weight loss by reducing the amount of circulating chemical toxins.

A recent article appearing in the *Journal of Alternative and Complementary Medicine* took an interesting look at chemical toxins and obesity. The author presented a hypothesis about chemical toxins that explains the global obesity epidemic. He claimed that the commonly held causes of obesity—overeating and inactivity—do not, based on his research, explain the current obesity epidemic. Instead, he makes a case that the current levels of chemical toxins impact the body's natural weight control mechanisms and contribute to obesity. And knowing what we know about toxins, including heavy metals, they could easily be affecting these control mechanisms.

The graphic correlation between the rise in toxins and the obesity epidemic is also striking. It seems that the rise in environmental toxins correlates very closely with the rise in the number of overweight individuals. This could explain why some people gain weight very easily while others do not. Our knowledge of variations from one individual to the next could explain why this is the case. For example, some people can detoxify better than others. It's possible that obese individuals are poor detoxifiers of certain chemicals that alter metabolic rate. Evaluating obese versus non-obese people and checking their detoxification systems may reveal some important information.

TOXIC CHEMICALS AND OBESITY

Ever since I began in medicine, diet and lifestyle have been the main focus when it comes to the causative factors of obesity. This has been, and continues to be, the main direction taken by physicians, dieticians, and the latest best-selling weight-loss authors. The problem with this approach is that it is always in flux. One diet goes out while the next diet comes in; it's enough to make your head spin.

We've learned an enormous amount about the toxic chemicals in the environment and their effects on human health. Thanks to the Toxome Project and other studies that show a body burden of hundreds of chemical toxins, there is little doubt that we are toxic. Toxic metals, pesticides, solvents, plasticizers, dyes, hormones, medicines, and flavoring agents make up just a small part of the thousands of chemicals that surround us. Some of these toxic chemicals have now been directly linked to obesity. For example, we are aware that organochlorine pesticides are stored in fat cells throughout the body. But did you know that, in animal studies, organochlorine (dieldrin) nearly doubled the total body fat content of treated mice? In another study, the pesticide known as lindane also induced weight gain in mice. It seems that organochlorines stored in fatty tissue cause weight gain by interfering with a number of weight control mechanisms in the human body.

Organochlorine's can disrupt various hormones that control weight gain. For example, in a 2002 study appearing in *Toxicological Sciences*, researchers followed subjects placed on a calorie restricted diet. They measured organochlorine levels as the patients lost weight, as well as T3 (active thyroid hormone responsible for metabolism). The result was that, as the subjects lost weight, their organochlorine levels went up and T3 went down. This demonstrates that organochlorines can have an impact on metabolism, slowing it down and therefore inducing weight gain. We know that these pesticides and toxic chemicals can mimic various neurotransmitters, possibly creating an imbalance within the nervous system.

TOXIC CHEMICALS AND THE NERVOUS SYSTEM

Many weight loss drugs on the market affect the sympathetic nervous system. These drugs mimic the effects of various neurotransmitters (communicating chemicals within the nervous system). As a result, these drugs have the ability to tell various cells what to do. These sympathomimetic agents, as they are called, can be used as weight loss drugs. These drugs work by suppressing appetite and acting as stimulants (ephedrine is a sympathomimetic-drug that mimics the effects of the sympathetic nervous system).

The sympathetic nervous system is also used in moments of stress, where it triggers the flight or fight response. Once this system is stimulated, the digestive tract shuts down. This will reduce appetite and slow down digestion. Toxic chemicals such as organochlorine pesticides can have an impact on the communicating abilities of these neurotransmitters. For example, they can inhibit their production, or interfere with their communicating abilities by blocking the lines of communications. These interactions can impact the sympathetic nervous system. The result? Obesity.

GROWTH PROMOTERS

Another aspect that is often overlooked is the impact that various chemicals and growth factors given to livestock have on human heath. We live in an era when chickens, beef, and other animals are fed a variety of products to help fatten them so they can be "market ready" in the least amount of time possible. These compounds are absorbed by the animals and are incorporated into the animal proteins and fats.

In the past, we've worried about the hormones found in these animals. But there are other chemicals and growth agents given to these animals that may also be affecting human health. The chemicals often found in livestock raised for food include anti-thyroid drugs (that slow down metabolism), corticosteroids, anabolic steroids, organophosphate pesticides, and carbamates.

WHAT HAVE WE LEARNED?

In this chapter we have begun to look at the real possibility that environmental toxins play an important role in obesity. There is little argument that these toxins exist and have penetrated our defenses, becoming a part of our physiology. Also, we see a remarkable parallel between the increase in obesity and the increase in our exposure to chemical toxins. This correlation is a starting point for our investigation. Evidence points to this strong connection and we must push further to confirm the validity of this connection. It could have a huge impact on the health of this nation.

12

CHAPTER TWELVE

Putting it All Together

BY NOW YOU SHOULD HAVE A fairly good idea that the world is a very toxic place. There isn't a square inch of land that hasn't been contaminated by one of the 85,000 registered man-made chemicals. The fact is, humans have created more environmental damage in the last 100 years than our ancestors have in thousands of years of civilization.

As the environmental movement continues to try to save our planet from contamination, health care providers must also try to protect human health from these same contaminants. We need to start by implementing strategies that will lessen our overall body burden. The Toxome Project has given us a glimpse into the startling reality that every human being is toxic.

Our goal now is to create and execute practical, effective strategies that can reduce this body burden. There are two ways of doing this. The first is to minimize toxic exposure and the second is to improve our body's ability to get rid of toxic chemicals.

THE PLAN
One of the main questions I get asked after giving patients the bad news about the level of toxins in their body is, "What do I do?" The goal of this chapter is to give you a framework that you can follow in

order to answer this important question. I'll break this down into four sections for simplicity and explain clearly how to go about following through with these directives.

Whole body cleansing involves two parts:

1. A daily regimen to help reduce overall exposure and enhance detoxification pathways called the **daily purification and prevention approach**.

2. A cleansing program that loosens bound toxins and eliminates them safely by supporting detoxification pathways (to be done three times per year) called the **whole body cleansing system.**

THE PROGRAM

One of the main issues I've had with most unscientific detoxification programs is the claim that these twice yearly kits are suppose to "do it all." We are exposed to toxins 24 hours a day and our bodies carry hundreds of these chemicals in various tissues. To assume that we can get these microscopic entities out of our systems by doing a kit once or twice a year is simply not realistic.

You can't get rid of lodged chemicals just by taking herbs mixed in a capsule and some fiber. Toxins need to be moved and then the body, through its own complex set of enzymes, needs to neutralize and remove them safely and effectively. Proper scientific detoxification involves the whole body cleansing approach which is made up of two parts.

The first part is a daily regimen that you need to incorporate into your life, starting now. I've put this in place because being successful in anything requires certain types of habitual behaviors. Achieving a reduced body burden also needs actions that are carried out daily. This includes incorporating a diet that will help you reduce toxic exposure and support your body's detoxification mechanisms. Remember, one of the biggest exposures is through the foods we consume, so it makes sense to assure the food you consume is as toxic free as possible. This can be accomplished by eating organically-grown foods whenever possible.

There are also foods that can help improve your overall detoxification mechanisms—antioxidants, fruits and vegetables, and that very important detoxification ingredient, dietary fiber. Adding these compounds to your daily diet will greatly enhance your ability to reduce overall body burden.

The second part of the Whole Body Cleansing approach is the detoxification phase. This involves taking certain supplements, restricting certain food items, and loosening toxins through infrared sauna or dry sauna. This is a three week program that is structured in such a way as to create a safe and effective means of clearing chemicals from the body. The concepts utilized are scientific and are evidence based.

DAILY PURIFICATION AND PREVENTION APPROACH

The Daily Purification and Prevention Approach is geared towards reducing overall exposure and enhancing detoxification mechanisms. This means becoming aware of chemical exposure from food, personal care products, and household cleaning agents. You must also become knowledgeable about the water you are drinking.

Last but not least you need to supplement the diet with nutrients that can help support your body's own detoxification systems. The best place to get these nutrients is from a high quality diet. This not only ensures optimal nutrition, but it also helps you ingest elements that can aid in detoxification and promote proper digestion. Very few people spend much time designing a diet that can help them achieve optimal health. Instead, they waste their time with weight loss diets, which eventually become weight gain diets.

A high quality diet means incorporating plenty of fresh organically-grown fruits and vegetables. It also means consuming less processed food that is free of preservatives, artificial dyes, and flavoring agents. A healthy diet means reducing your consumption of sugar and consuming more complex carbohydrates. In addition, you should eat less meat and, when you do, make sure it's hormone-free, organically-grown meat. Don't forget that consuming healthy fish and plenty of pure water completes a healthy diet.

THE 6 KEYS TO A HEALTHY DIET:

- Consume organically-grown fresh fruits and vegetables daily.
- Reduce meat consumption and make sure the meat you eat is certified organic.
- Eat fish with the least amount of toxic metals.
- Reduce unhealthy fats and increase essential fatty acids.
- Include plenty of dietary fiber—40 grams total per day.
- Drink at least eight 8-ounce glasses of water per day.

10 STEPS TO REDUCE YOUR OVERALL EXPOSURE AND ENHANCE DETOXIFICATION MECHANISMS

1. Eat organically-grown fruits and vegetables.

Don't be misled by people who assume that the advantage of eating organic fruits and vegetable is nutritional value. This isn't the reason I recommend them. The reason to eat organic fruits and vegetables is to reduce toxic chemical exposure. Certified organic fruits and vegetables are free from pesticides and other chemical sprays. Remember that, in the United States alone, over one billion pounds of pesticides are sprayed and added to food crops each year. If you do your math, that translates to about four pounds for every man, woman, and child in the United States. We need to get away from this type of exposure and organic produce seems to be the answer.

As we all know, consuming fresh fruits and vegetables also has tremendous health benefits that are supported by almost every government agency. Even the American Cancer Society recommends the consumption of fruit and vegetables for the prevention of cancer. Fruits and vegetables also contain a number of antioxidants and phytochemicals that support detoxification mechanisms.

If you can't afford to buy organically-grown fruits and vegetables, or if they are not available in your area, you can make some adjustments. Peel, clean, and brush the fruits and vegetables to remove at least some of the chemical residue.

2. Reduce meat consumption and switch to organically-raised meat when you do indulge.

One of the biggest problems with the American diet is the high consumption of meat. Conventionally-grown animal foods have been linked to heart disease, cancer, and obesity. There are a number of reasons why this is so, but we'll focus on the two main ones. First, meat products—which include beef, pork, chicken, and turkey—contain high levels of arachadonic acid. The typical Western diet contains far too much arachadonic acid and not enough omega-3 fatty acids like EPA and DHA. High levels of arachadonic acid can lead to high levels of inflammation in the body which can ultimately contribute to a host of health problems. Reducing arachadonic acid levels by reducing the consumption of these meats can lower overall inflammation in the body.

The second problem with meat is the way the animals are raised. Most conventionally-raised livestock are fed hormones, steroids, antibiotics, and other growth factors to promote rapid development and fattening in order to get the animals to market in a shorter period of time. There is a high probability that these drugs are passed on to consumers to some degree. In essence, we are exposing ourselves to a number of hormones including xenoestrogens (substances that act like estrogen in the body) with every hamburger, steak or pork chop. Switching to certified organic meats will not only improve your health but it will reduce your chemical exposure. If you can't afford to purchase organic meat, try to eliminate meat altogether or greatly reduce your consumption.

3. Consume fish with minimal toxic metal levels.

Our oceans and major lakes are highly polluted—and so are the fish that live in them. Many fish have been contaminated with mercury, PCBs, and other toxic substances. As mentioned earlier much of the tuna sold in your local supermarket contains large amounts of mercury that can easily be incorporated into the human body after being eaten. To learn which fish are healthy to consume in your area visit the Monterey Bay Aquarium website for information about the toxicity levels in fish, as well as issues regarding sustainability (www.montereybayaquarium.org).

As a rule of thumb, it's wise to consume fish that have been caught in water that has not been contaminated by industrial waste. Healthy fish are wild salmon, halibut, and some types of cod. Many large predatory fish like tuna, swordfish, rockfish, orange roughy, and Chilean seabass contain high levels of mercury. Farmed salmon contain PCBs. Minimizing your exposure to these fish will help reduce your body's toxin levels.

4. Consume healthy fats.

As we discussed earlier, consuming essential fatty acids, like those found in fish, is important. These important fats are incorporated into cell membranes, improving overall cell function. Having cells function optimally is an important step in creating optimal health.

Supplementing the diet with good omega-3 oils, especially EPA and DHA found in fish, is a great way to achieve balance. At the same time, it's important to reduce your overall consumption of saturated fats and trans-fats from meat, margarine, shortening, and other foods that contain hydrogenated oils. Start using healthy fats like coconut oil for cooking and olive oil for salads instead.

Note: If you can, use triglyceride based fish oils such as Eskimo-3 or some Nordic Natural products.

5. Consume 40 grams of dietary fiber per day.

I won't spend a lot of the time on fiber since I discussed it at length in earlier chapters. But dietary fiber is a critical component in your daily diet. Fiber will never get absorbed by your body. Instead it acts like a transient visitor who does a wonderful job of cleaning you up and leaving you better off than when it came in.

Fiber, including both soluble and insoluble fiber, can have a number of benefits that include blood sugar regulation, cholesterol lowering effects, improving stool transit time, and preventing constipation. By taking fiber daily, you will also support detoxification mechanisms as well.

Increasing your fruit and vegetable consumption will automatically increase the amount of fiber in your diet. To make sure you are getting more than enough of this critical nutrient, take a powdered fiber supplement at night and again in the morning.

My favorite is Fiber Fusion by Enzymatic Therapy, which is available in powder form or as capsules.

Note: Another excellent fiber is called PGX and also available at leading health food stores.

6. Include at least eight 8-ounce glasses of purified water daily.

Science tells us that the human body is anywhere from 55 to 75 percent water, depending on body size. To function properly, you need to replace the water lost through sweat and urination on a daily basis. Although our recommendation is for eight 8-ounce glasses of water per day, the precise amount depends on the level of activity, temperature, humidity, and other factors.

This seems like a simple thing to do but many people have a difficult time with it. The typical reason is because they don't actually feel thirsty, but, once they start drinking water, they find that they do develop a thirst. But it's important to make sure the water you drink is pure and not contaminated. Try using a filtration system in your home or purchase bottled water that is certified pure by independent analysis. As I mentioned earlier, Fiji water is one of several brands that clearly indicates where their water comes from and has an analysis of its purity on their web site.

7. Make sure you get seven to eight hours of sleep per night.

Sleep is a very important part of overall health. Yet, too often, we assume that being sleep deprived just makes us tired the next day. But the reality is very different from this assumption. It turns out that not getting seven to eight hours of sleep per night can have some serious health consequences. In a landmark study at the University of Chicago, researchers found that people that slept 6.5 hours or less had a 50 percent increase in the insulin blood levels compared to those that slept 7.5 to 8.5 hours per night. This not only puts people at risk for developing Type II diabetes but can also contribute to obesity.

Making sure that you get your eight hours of sleep each night will ensure optimally functioning physiology and improved detoxification. If you are not sleeping properly, find out what the problem is. Elevated cortisol or some other hormonal imbalance could be at the root of your sleep problems. One product I recommend is Sleep Tonight that dramatically lowers cortisol. This product has a number of calming ingredients that include ashwagandha, magnolia officinalis, epimedium, L-theanine and phosphatidylserine. ProSleep is another product that lulls you to sleep.

8. Supplements.

There are a number of supplements you should add to your daily regimen to support the body. A multivitamin-mineral complex is something I recommend to my patients because it is an essential part of a healthy diet. Studies show that a multivitamin-mineral supplement provides concrete health benefits, regardless of what some mainstream folks might be saying.

Probiotics are also turning out to be more important than anyone thought. Studies show many different benefits in gastrointestinal function. Keeping your GI tract healthy is a key process in detoxification.

PROBIOTICS: Take a probiotic supplement daily before bedtime. Make sure it has a minimum of two species of bacteria, *Lactobacillus acidophilus* and *Bifidobacterium longum*. Also, when choosing a probiotic, make sure it's stable at room temperature and provides guaranteed delivery to the gut at the time of purchase.

MULTIVITAMIN-MINERAL COMPLEX: A good multivitamin-mineral complex is something everyone should take daily. An excellent multivitamin-mineral with antioxidants is the Alive brand, available in most grocery outlets and health food stores.

OMEGA-3 FISH OILS: Triglyceride-based fish oil supplying about a gram of fish oil per capsule is what I often recommend to my patients. Triglyceride oils are in their natural form and seem to be more stable as supplements. As mentioned earlier this type of oil can be found in brands like Eskimo-3 and Nordic Naturals.

9. Opt for natural personal care products.

Take a look at the grooming products you use every day—soap, toothpaste, deodorant, shampoo, moisturizer, and shaving cream. Each one of these products contains chemicals that, over a period of time, can accumulate in your body. You can easily replace all of them with more naturally-based personal care products that don't contain carcinogenic and endocrine-disrupting chemicals like plasticizers and preservatives.

Go to your local health food store and ask for replacements for each one of these products. You'll be surprised at the wide array of options. As a bonus, your skin will look and feel much better after you switch.

10. Change the cleaning agents in your home.

Home is where the toxins are. As we learned earlier, the inside of your home can be 25 to 100 times more toxic than the outside. Although there are a lot of sources of pollutants inside a home, there are definite cost effective steps you can take to minimize this exposure.

Some areas you may not be able to do anything about are carpets and paint. Most carpets emit nearly 200 toxic chemicals and studies on carpet installers show that these individuals have issues with the chemicals they are being exposed to. If you need to replace your carpeting, think of installing carpet made from natural fibers free of toxic chemicals.

If you decide you want to change the colors of your home, choose a VOC-free paint. Many paint companies are now making natural paints with minimal toxic elements. This is definitely a move in the right direction.

One thing you can change immediately are the cleaning products you use. Dish soap, cleaning agents, laundry detergents, herbicides and pesticides, and oven cleaners all contain chemicals that are circulating in your home and become incorporated into your body. You can change this by switching to environmentally-friendly products that are void of toxic chemicals. Most major grocery stores now carry green cleaning products.

One other source of toxins you may not be aware of are the chemicals that are released by your non-stick pans. One of the Toxome studies looked at perfluorooctane sulfonate (PFOS) and found it in the umbilical cords of new born infants. Also found in microwave popcorn, PFOS's can cause some serious problems.

THE 3-WEEK WHOLE BODY CLEANSING SYSTEM
(TO BE PRACTICED TWO TO THREE TIMES PER YEAR.)

In all of the detoxification discussions I've had with my patients, probably the most important topic that comes up is what kind of program they should engage in. There are so many different programs available and my patients usually want to know which one actually works. The truth is, however, that most of these programs fail to deliver on their promises because they aren't based on science.

I've put together a program that will give you results by dislodging the toxic chemicals in your body. These toxins are then neutralized and bound in a safe and effective manner for excretion. My complete detoxification program is a three week plan that should be repeated three times per year. During the first week, you'll be preparing for the full detox while increasing the antioxidant levels in the body. You'll be restricting your diet and reducing as much toxic exposure as possible. Weeks two and three will be the start of the actual detoxification process. Toxins will be loosened and, with help from the recommended supplement program, you will bind and excrete a majority of them toxins.

WEEK 1 – PREPARATION PHASE

Purpose:
- Preparation for Weeks 2 and 3.
- Increasing body antioxidant levels through diet and supplementation.
- Eliminating processed foods, alcohol, and caffeine.

Background:
During the preparation phase you will need to restrict the amount of food you eat and completely eliminate certain foods and beverages (see Table 12.1). The idea is to minimize the workload your GI tract and liver have to do and thus give them plenty of energy to deal with detoxification mechanisms.

Juicing has been popularized by all sorts of television shows and juicing machines are now available in most department and discount stores. It is an excellent way to get enzymes, phytochemicals, vitamins, and minerals into your system in high concentrations. The fresh juice recipe I recommend is easy to make and the ingredients are readily available. Drink this either in the morning or with dinner. It will provide antioxidants and phytochemicals that can help increase your antioxidant load to help your body handle the chemicals that will be released in week 3 and 4.

Drink 6 ounces of pomegranate juice daily for the entire 3 weeks. Pomegranate juice (I recommend POM Wonderful) contains ellagic acid, a phenolic compound with great detoxification properties.

Supplements provide nutrients that are sometimes difficult to get from your diet. The supplement I recommend for this phase is called Whole Body Multivitamin Cleanse (available in natural health stores), also known as Detoxification Factors (for healthcare professionals). This product has a number of vitamins and antioxidants that can greatly aid in the detoxification processes.

Every night, you'll drink about two to three 8-ounce glasses of water, each with the juice of one-half squeezed lemon. This is an excellent way to increase your hydration levels. Not only does the lemon provide flavor, it adds some extra vitamin C.

Summary for Week 1 (Monday-Sunday)

- Whole Body Multivitamin Cleanse or Detoxification Factors, 2 capsules with lunch.
- Rencancostat, 1 teaspoon added to juice taken once daily.
- Juice, every morning (2 carrots, ½ apple, 1 orange, handful of parsley, ½ beet; add 1 teaspoon of rencancostat).
- Night – Two to three 8-ounce glasses of water with ½ lemon.

TABLE 12.1   DIETARY RESTRICTIONS FOR WEEK 1 TO 3

Dietary Restriction for Preparation and Detoxification For 3-Week Program	
Things to Avoid	Thing That Can Replace
Alcohol, coffee, soft drinks, hot chocolate	Water, sparkling water, herbal teas
Refined carbohydrates found in cakes, cookies, muffins, donuts, ice cream, etc.	Foods sweetened with stevia
Artificial sweeteners, table sugar	Stevia
No chemical additives, preservatives, dyes, coloring agents, flavors, etc.	Unprocessed foods
Meats, chicken, pork, turkey, processed meats, hot dogs, etc.	Small servings (3 oz.) of organic meat; wild salmon
Fried food, trans fats	Coconut oil, omega-3, olive oil for salads.

WEEK 2 AND 3 – DETOXIFICATION AND TOXIN DISLODGING PHASE

Purpose:
- Dislodge chemical toxins from various tissues around the body.
- To eliminate these toxins in a safe and effective manner by improving detoxification mechanisms.
- Elimination of processed foods, including alcohol and caffeine.

Background:
You will continue the diet you adopted during Week 1. This will continue to help your liver and digestive tract cope with the large amounts of chemicals you'll be releasing into the blood stream.

Utilizing the infra-red sauna every other day will help dislodge chemicals. Infra-red penetrates into the adipose tissue, where it begins to loosen bound toxins. This should be done every other day for about 40 minutes; you can increase it to one hour maximum if you can tolerate it. Make sure you drink plenty of water while in the sauna to stay hydrated. If you have high blood pressure or other medical conditions, check with your doctor before adding this step.

If you don't have access to an infrared sauna, you can achieve similar effects by exercising intensively for about 60 minutes per day. This can be accomplished by working on a treadmill or a stationary bike, or even hiking your favorite trail. The idea here is to get into fat burning mode which will help release toxins.

Once toxins are dislodged, you want to begin binding through Phase I and II detoxification mechanisms and then through the GI tract for elimination. This will entail taking certain supplements that can help you achieve these effects.

The phase will take a total of 14 days to complete.

The supplements you'll take during these two weeks include a Whole Body Cleanse kit that contains fiber component, a laxative based on magnesium hydroxide, and a liver component based on milk thistle. All of these supplements were discussed in Chapter 7.

During Week 3, I also recommend Whole Body Liver Cleanse which provides high levels of liver-specific antioxidants and Calcium-D-glucarate to improve glucoronidation reactions.

DIM (diindolylmethane) is a product that should also be added, 2 capsules per day. This will help your body deal with the high levels of xenoestrogens being released.

Summary

Product		Week 2	Week 3	Purpose
Whole Body Cleanse	Fiber component	4 capsules in morning, 4 capsules at night	4 capsules in morning, 4 capsules at night	Insures proper soluble fiber levels to bind bile
	Liver Formula	2 capsules in morning, 2 capsules at night	1 capsule in morning, 1 capsule at night	Helps support Phase I and II detoxification
	Laxative	2 tablets at night	2 tablets at night	Increases bowel movements
Whole Body Liver Cleanse			2 capsules morning, 1 capsule at night	Specific liver support formula
DIM		2 tablets daily	2 tablets daily	Supports the elimination of xenoestrogens
Whole Body Multivitamin		2 capsules daily	2 capsules daily	Supports Phase I and II reactions
Recancostat 400		2 capsules	2 capsules	Supplies glutathione

FINAL THOUGHTS

I remember when I was a young boy listening to my parents talking about a family friend who was in the hospital with a serious illness. I recall them saying something that I've heard many times since, "Your health is everything." How many of us believe that this is true and even more importantly how many of us let our actions reflect that belief? It seems that many of us would rather spend money tuning up our vehicles than tuning up our bodies. It is my hope and dream that after reading this book, you begin the process. Start making the necessary changes and continue learning about your health.

The purpose of this book is to help you achieve better health by removing the chemical toxins—the obstacles—that impede the body's innate ability to heal itself. There is little doubt that we live in a toxic world, one where chemicals have infiltrated every square inch of space. These chemicals inhabit the air we breathe, the food we eat, the water we drink and even the things that come in contact with our skin. In other words they are ubiquitous, found everywhere and in everything. These facts should be all that is needed to change our views about how to improve our health.

Our focus should be on reducing our exposure to the numerous chemical toxins that are found in every aspect of our lives. These are the chemicals that have been a health hazard for decades, yet only now—after years of denial—has the scientific community begun to look at how they are affecting human physiology. What we know and can assume is that they can affect almost every aspect of cellular function including our precious genetics. This can have far reaching consequences with enormous impact on general human health. It may be the reason why so many new diseases are appearing and so many old ones continue to plague us.

There is little doubt that we need to minimize our exposure to environmental toxins and, at the same time, enhance our body's own ability to get rid of them. This can be accomplished by having a greater understanding of what is going on environmentally and then starting to follow the simple plan laid out in this chapter. It is a scientific and safe way of reducing your overall toxic burden and beginning your journey to wellness. The body has an innate ability to heal itself, given the right environment. By following this plan, you will be taking the first steps on the road to achieving optimal health.

REFERENCES BY CHAPTER

Introduction

Broad Scan Analysis of the FY82 National Human Adipose Tissue Survey Specimens. EPA Office of Toxic Substances. EPA-560/5-86-035.

Hayes T, Haston K, Tsui M, et al. Feminization of male frogs in the wild. *Nature*. 419: 895-896, 2002.

Lawson L. *Staying Well in a Toxic World*. Chicago: The Nobel Press Inc., 1993.

Perera FP. Molecular Epidemiology: Insights into Cancer Susceptibility, Risk Assessment, and Prevention. *Journal of the National Cancer Institute*. 88: 496-509, 1996.

Perera FP, Rauh V, Tsai WY, et al. Effects of transplacental exposure to environmental pollutants on birth outcomes in a multi-ethnic population. *Environmental Health Perspectives*. 111:201-206, 2003.

Pizzorno JE, Murray MT. *A Textbook of Natural Medicine*. 2nd Ed. London: Churchill Livingstone, 1999.

Watters E. DNA Is Not Destiny. *Discover Magazine*. 75:32-37, November 2006.

Chapter 1

Colborn T, Dumanoski, D, Myers JP. *Our Stolen Future*. New York: Dutton, 1996.

Nick GL. *Clinical Purification: A Complete Treatment and Reference Manual*. Brookfield, Wisconsin: Longevity Through Prevention Books. 2001:167-178,

Roundtree R. The Use of Phytochemicals in the Biotransformation and Elimination of Environmental Toxins. *Medicines from the Earth 2003: Official Proceedings.* Gaia Herbal Research Institute. Brevard, NC 115-128, 2003.

Chapter 2

Afshari A, Gunnarsen L, Clausen PA, et al. Emission of phthalates from PVC and other material. *Indoor Air.* 14:120–128, 2004.

Brock JW, Caudill SP, Silva MJ, et al. Phthalate monoesters levels in the urine of young children. *Bulletin of Environmental Contamination and Toxicology.* 68:309–314, 2002.

Burt T. Sick Building Syndrome: Acoustic Aspects. *Indoor and Built Environment.* 5: 44-59. 1996.

EWG/Commonweal Study #4, Industrial chemicals and pesticides in cord blood. Health effects of pollutants found in people. Human Toxome Project. Available at www.ewg.org/sites/humantoxome/healtheffects.

Hauser R, Calafat AM. Phthalates and human health; *Occupational and Environmental Medicine.* 62:806-818, 2005.

Wallace LA, Pellizzari ED, Hartwell TD, et al. The TEAM (Total Exposure Assessment Methodology) Study: personal exposures to toxic substances in air, drinking water, and breath of 400 residents of New Jersey, North Carolina, and North Dakota. *Environmental Research.* 143:290–307, 1987.

Wormuth M, Scheringer M, Vollenweider M, What are the sources of exposure to eight frequently used phthalic acid esters in Europeans? *Risk Analysis.* 26:803–824, 2006.

Chapter 3

A Poison Kiss: The Problem of Lead in Lipsticks, The Campaign for Safe Cosmetics, 2007. Available at www.safecosmetics.org.

Beseler CL, Stallones L, Hoppin JA, et al. Depression and pesticide exposure among private pesticide applicators enrolled in the Agricultural Health Study. *Environmental. Health Perspectives.* 116:1713–1719, 2008.

Clark S, Menrath W, Chen M, et al. The influence of exterior dust and soil lead on interior dust lead levels in housing that had undergone lead-based paint hazard control. *Journal of Occupational and Environmental Hygiene.* 1: 273–282, 2004.

Cordes DH, Foster D. Health hazards of farming. *American Family Physician.* 38: 233–244, 1988.

Daniels JL, Olshan AF, Savitz DA. Pesticides and childhood cancers. *Environmerntal. Health Perspectives.* 105: 1068–1077, 1997.

Ecobichon DJ. *Casarett and Doull's Toxicology: The Basic Science of Poisons.* 5th ed. New York: MacMillan, 643–689, 1996.

ECSCF. Opinion of the Scientific Committee on Food on Bisphenol A. SCF/CS/ PM/ 3936 Final. Brussels: European Commission Scientific Committee on Food, 2002. Available: http://europa.eu.int/comm/food/fs/sc/scf/out128_en.pdf.

The National Water Quality Inventory: Report for Congress fro the 2002 Registry Cycle- A Profile. Fact Sheet No. EPA 841-F-07-003, Environmental Protection Agency (EPA), Washington, D.C. October 2007.

Eskenazi B, Bradman A, Castorina R. Exposure of children to organophosphate pesticides and their potential adverse health effects. *Environmental Health Perspectives.* 107: 409–419, 1999.

Jaga K, Dharmani C. Sources of exposure to and public health implications of organophosphate pesticides. *Revista panamericana de Salud Publica.* 14: 171–185, 2003.

Jarup L, Berglund M, Elinder CG, et al. Health effects of cadmium exposure—a review of the literature and a risk estimate. *Scandinavian Journal of Work, Environment and Health* 24: 11–51, 1998.

Klaasen CD, and John Doull. *Casarett and Doull's Toxicology: The Basic Science of Poisons,* 6th ed. New York: McGraw Hill, 2001.

Mackert JR. Dental amalgam and mercury. *Journal of the American Dental Association.* 122:54-61, 1991.

Mackert JR Jr, Berglund A. Mercury exposure from dental amalgam fillings absorbed dose and the potential for adverse health effects. *Critical Review of Oral Biology and Medicine.* 8:410-436, 1997.

Most Bottled Water Brands Don't Disclose Information About Source, Purity and Contaminants. Environmental Working Group (EWG), Washington, D.C. 2009.

Nogawa K, Kobayashi E, Okubo Y, et al. Environmental cadmium exposure, adverse effects and preventative measures in Japan. *Biometals.* 17: 581–587, 2004.

Rogers SA. Chemical Sensitivity: Breaking the Paralyzing Paradigm. *Internal Medicine World Report.* 7:15-16, 1992.

Tang N, Zhu ZQ, Adverse reproductive effects in female workers of lead battery plants. *International Journal of Occupational Medicine and Environmental Health,* 16:359-361, 2003.

Toxic Air Pollutants. Environmental Protection Agency, Washington, D.C., April 2009.

Wallace LA, Pellizzari ED, Hartwell TD, et al. Personal exposures, indoor-outdoor relationships, and breath levels of toxic air pollutants measured for 355 persons in New Jersey. *Atmospheric Environment.* 19:1651-1661, 1985.

Yassin A S, Martonik JF. Urinary cadmium levels in the U.S. working population, 1988–1994. *Journal of Occupational and Environmental Hygiene.* 1: 324–333, 2004.

Chapter 4

Broughton A, Thrasher JD. Chronic health effects and immunological alterations associated with exposure to pesticides. *Common Toxicology.* 4:59-71, 1990.

Colborn T, vom Saal FS, Soto AM. Developmental effects of endocrine-disrupting chemicals in wildlife and humans. *Environmental Health Perspectives.* 101: 378–384, 1993.

Cooper GP, Manalis RS. Influence of heavy metals on synaptic transmission: a review. *Neurotoxicology* 4:69-83, 1983.

Golden RJ, Noller KL, Titus-Ernstoff L, et al. Environmental endocrine modulators and human health: an assessment of the biological evidence. *Critical Reviews in Toxicology.* 28: 109–227, 1998.

Hayes T, Haston K, Tsui M, et al. Atrazine-Induced Hermaphroditism at 0.1 PPB in American Leopard Frogs (*Rana pipiens*): Laboratory and Field Evidence. *Environmental Health Perspectives.* 111:568-575, 2003.

Hueser G. Diagnostic markers in clinical immunotoxicology and neurotoxicology. *Journal of Occupational Medicine and Toxicology.* 1:5-9, 1992.

Kiesecker JM. Synergism between trematode infection and pesticide exposure: A link to amphibian limb deformities in nature? *Proceedings of the National Academy of Sciences.* 99: 9900-9904, 2002.

Lieb J, Hershman D. Isaac Newton: mercury poisoning or manic depression. *Lancet.* 2:1479-1480, 1983.

Lottrup G, Andersson AM, Leffers H, et al. Possible impact of phthalates on infant reproductive health. *International Journal of Andrology*. 29:172–180, 2006.

Luster MI, Rosenthal GJ. Chemical agents and the immune response. *Environmental Health Perspectives*. 100:219-226, 1993.

Luster MI, Rosenthal GJ. The Immunosuppressive influence of industrial and environmental xenobiotics. *TIPS*. 408-412, 1986.

McPherson JD, Shilton BH, Walton DJ. Role of fructose in glycation and cross-linking of proteins. *Biochemistry*. 27:1901-1907, 1988.

Melpomeni P, Uribarri J, Vlassara H. Glucose, advanced glycation end products, and diabetes complications: What is new and what works. *Clinical Diabetes*. 21:,186-187, 2003.

Ngim CH, Foo SC, Boey KW, et al. Chronic neurobehaviorual effects of elemental mercury in dentists. *British Journal of Industrial Medicine*. 49:782-790, 1992.

Ninomiya T, Ohmori H, Hashimoto K, et al. Expansion of methylmercury poisoning outside of Minamata: epidemiological study on chronic methylmercury poisoning outside Minamata. *Environmental Research*. 70:47-50, 1995.

Perera, FP. Environment and cancer: who are susceptible? *Science*. 278:1068-1073, 1997.

Porth CM. Lymphatic system. Pathophysiology. In *Concepts of Altered Health States*. 5th ed. Philadelphia, PA: Lippincott. 427-428, 2002.

Quesada I, Fuentes E, Viso-Leon MC, et al. Low doses of the endocrine disruptor bisphenol-A and the native hormone 17-beta-estradiol rapidly activate transcription factor CREB. *FASEB Journal*. 16:1671-1673, 2002.

Rattan S. Theories of biological aging: genes, proteins, and free radicals. *Free Radical Research*. 40: 1230–1238, 2006.

Rea WJ. *Chemical Sensitivity* Vol. 3. Boca Raton, FL: CRC Press, 1996.

Schettler T, Solomon G, Valenti M, et al. *Generations at Risk: Reproductive Health and the Environment*. Cambridge, MA: MIT Press, 1999.

Selgrade MK, Cooper GS, Germolec DR, et al. Linking environmental agents to autoimmune disease. *Environmental Health Perspectives*. 107:S5811-S811, 1999.

Sohal R, Mockett R, Orr W. Mechanisms of aging: an appraisal of the oxidative stress hypothesis. *Free Radical Biology & Medicine*. 33: 575–586, 2002.

Sohal R. Role of oxidative stress and protein oxidation in the aging process. *Free Radical Biology & Medicine*. 33: 37–44, 2002.

Solomon GM, Schettler T. Environment and health: Endocrine disruption and potential human health implications. *CMAJ* 163: 1471–1476, 2000.

Swan SH, Main KM, Liu F, et al. Decrease in anogenital distance among male infants with prenatal phthalate exposure. *Environmental Health Perspectives*. 113:1056–1061, 2005.

Vial T, Nicolas B, Descotes J. Clinical immunotoxicity of pesticides. *Journal of Toxicology and Environmental Health*. 48:215-229, 1996.

Vlassara H. Advanced glycation in health and disease: Role of the modern environment. *Annals of the New York Academy of Science*. 1043: 452–460, 2005.

Vojdani A, Ghoneum M, Brautbar N. Immune alteration associated with exposure to toxic chemicals. *Toxicology and Industrial Health*. 8:239-253, 1992.

Vial T, Nicolas B, Descotes J. Clinical Immunotoxicity of Pesticides. *Journal of Toxicology and Environmental Health* 48:215-229, 1996.

Watters E. DNA Is Not Destiny. *Discover Magazine*. 75:32-37, November 2006.

Chapter 5

Bandmann O, Vaughan J, Holmans P, et al. Association of slow acetylator genotype for Nacetyltransferase 2 with familial Parkinson's disease. *Lancet*. 1350:1136-1139, 1997.

Beckett GJ, Hayes JD. Glutathione S-transferases: biomedical applications. *Advances in Clinical Chemistry*. 30: 281–380, 1993.

Beckett GJ, Hayes JD. Glutathione S-transferase measurements and liver disease in man. *Journal of Clinical Biochemistry and Nutrition*. 2: 1–24, 1987.

Daly AK, Cholerton S, Gregory W, Idle J. Metabolic polymorphisms. *Pharmacology & Therapeutics*. 57:129-160, 1993.

Estabrook RW. Cytochrome P450: From a single protein to a family of proteins—with some personal reflections. In *Cytochromes P450: Metabolic And Toxicological Aspects*. Boca Raton, FL: CRC Press, Inc. 3-28, 1996.

Feldman EB. How grapefruit juice potentiates drug bioavailability. *Nutrition Review*. 55:398-400, 1997.

Fuhr U, Klittich K, Staib H. Inhibitory effect of grapefruit juice and its bitter principal, naringenin, on CYP1A2 dependent metabolism of caffeine in man. *British Journal of Clinical Pharmacology.* 35:431-436, 1993.

Guengerich FP. Effects of nutritive factors on metabolic processes involving bioactivation and detoxification of chemicals. *Annual Review of Nutrition.* 4:207-231, 1984.

Guengerich FP. Influence of nutrients and other dietary materials on cytochrome P450 enzymes. *American Journal of Clinical Nutrition.* 61 (3 Suppl): 651S-658S, 1995.

Hutt AJ, Caldwell J. Amino acid conjugation. *Conjugation Reactions In Drug Metabolism.* New York: Taylor & Francis. 273-305, 1990.

Kall MA, Clausen J. Dietary effect on mixed function P450 1A2 activity assayed by estimation of caffeine metabolism in man. *Human & Experimental Toxicology.* 14:801-807, 1995.

Manson MM, Ball HWL, Barrett MC, et al. Mechanism of action of dietary chemoprotective agents in rat liver: induction of phase I and II drug metabolizing enzymesand aflatoxin B1 metabolism. *Carcinogenesis.* 18:1729-1738, 1997.

Meyer UA, Zanger UM, Skoda RC, et al. Genetic polymorphisms of drug metabolism. *Progress in Liver Disease.* 9:307-323, 1990.

Pizzorno JE, Murray MT. *A Textbook of Natural Medicine*, 2nd Ed. London: Churchill Livingstone, 1999.

Roundtree R. The use of phytochemicals in the biotransformation and elimination of environmental toxins. *Medicines from the Earth 2003: Official Proceedings.* Gaia Herbal Research Institute, Brevard, N.C. 115-128, 2003.

Slattery JT, Wilson JM, Kalhorn TF, et al. Dose-dependent pharmacokinetics of acetaminophen: Evidence of glutathione depletion in humans. *Clinical Pharmacology and Therapeutics.* 41:413-418, 1987.

Spatzenegger M, Jaeger W. Clinical importance of hepatic cytochrome P450 in drug metabolism. *Drug Metabolism Reviews.* 27:397-417, 1995.

Wacher VJ, Wu C-Y, Benet LZ. Overlapping substrate specificities and tissue distribution of cytochrome P450 3A and P-glycoprotein: Implications for drug delivery and activity in cancer chemotherapy. *Molecular Carcinogenesis.* 13:129-134, 1995.

Wilce MC, Parker MW. Structure and function of glutathione S-transferases. *Biochimica et biophysica acta.* 1205: 1–18, 1994.

Chapter 6

Bardhan KD, Cumberland DC, Dixon RA, et al. Clinical trial of deglycyrrhisinated liqourice in gastric ulcer. *Gut.* 19:779-782, 1978.

Bardnan KD, Cumberland DC, Dixon RA, et al. Proceedings: Deglycrrhizinated liqourice in gastric ulcer: a double-blind controlled trial. *Gut.* 17:397, 1976.

Dajani EZ, Klamut GMJ. Novel therapeutic approaches to gastric and duodenal ulcers: an update. *Expert Opinion on Investigational Drugs.* 9:1537-1544, 2000.

Dehpour AR, Zolfaghari ME, Sadian T, et al. The protective effect of liquorice components and their derivatives against gastric ulcer induced by aspirin in rats. *Journal of Pharmacy and Pharmacology.* 46:148-149, 1994.

Engqvist A, von Feilitzen F, Pyk E, et al Double-blind trial of deglycyrrhizinated liqourice in gastric ulcer. *Gut.* 14:711-715, 1973.

Galland L. Leaky Gut Syndromes: Breaking the Vicious Cycles. *Townsend Letter for Doctors.* August/September 1995.

Glick L. Deglycyrrhizinated liqourice for peptic ulcer. *Lancet.* 9:817, 1982.

Graham DY, Malaty HM. Alendronate and naproxen are synergistic for development of gastric ulcers. *Archives of Internal Medicine.* 161:107-110, 2001.

Hawkey CJ, Nonsteroidal anti-inflammatory drug gastropathy. *Gastroenterology.* 119:521-535, 2000.

Kiefer D, Ali-Akbarian L. A brief evidence-based review of two gastrointestinal illnesses: irritable bowel and leaky gut syndromes. *Alternative Therapies in Health and Medicine.* 10: 22–30, 2004.

Mitsuoska T. Intestinal flora and aging. *Nutrition Review.* 50:438-446, 1992.

Nick GL. The intestinal tract. In *Clinical Purification: A Complete Treatment and Reference Manual.* Brookfield, WI: Longevity Through Prevention Books, 2001.

Pizzorno, JE, Murray, MT. *Textbook of Natural Medicine*, 3rd edition. London: Churchill Livingstone. 2005:167, 584, 1527

Rees WDW, Rhodes J, Wright JE, et al. Effect of deglycyrrhizinated liqourice on gastric mucosal damage by aspirin. *Scandinavian Journal of Gastroenterology.* 14:605-607, 1979.

Scheline RR. Metabolism of foreign compounds by gastrointestinal microorganisms. *Pharmacology Review.* 25:451-523, 1973.

Smith MD, Gibson RA, Brooks PM. Abnormal bowel permeability in ankylosing spondylitis and rheumatoid arthritis. *Journal of Rheumatology.* 2:299-305, 1985.

Trolli PA. Pancreatic enzyme therapy and nutritional status of outpatients with chronic pancreatitis. *Gastroenterology Nursing.* 24:84-87, 2001.

Wollowski I, Rechkemmer G, Pool-Zobel BL. Protective role of probiotics and prebiotics in colon cancer. *American Journal of Clinical Nutrition.* 73:451S-455S, 2001.

Chapter 7

Anderson JW, Hanna TJ. Impact of nondigestible carbohydrates on serum lipoproteins and risk for cardiovascular disease. *Journal of Nutrition.* 129:1457S-66S, 1999.

Asai A, Miyazawa T. Dietary curcuminoids prevent high-fat diet-induced lipid accumulation in rat liver and epididymal adipose tissue. *Journal of Nutrition.* 131:2932-2935, 2001.

Ballatori N, Lieberman MW, Wang W. N-acetylcysteine as an antidote in methylmercury poisoning. *Environmental Health Perspectives.* 106:267-271, 1998.

Bandmann O, Vaughan J, Holmans P, et al. Association of slow acetylator genotype for Nacetyltransferase 2 with familial Parkinson's disease. *Lancet.* 350:1136-1139, 1997.

Bartter FC, Berkson BM, Gallelli J, et al. Treatment of Four Delayed-Mushroom-Poisoning Patients with Thioctic Acid. In *Amanita Toxins and Poisonings*, New York: Witzstrock, Baden-Baden, 1980.

Barzaghi N, Crema F, Gatti G, et al. Pharmacokinetic studies on IdB 1016, a silybinphosphatidylcholine complex, in healthy human subjects. *European Journal of Drug Metabolism and Pharmacokinetics.* 15:333-338, 1990.

Berkson, B. Thioctic acid in treatment of hepatotoxic mushroom poisoning (letter). *New England Journal of Medicine.* 300:371, 1979.

Berkson BM. A conservative triple antioxidant approach to the treatment of hepatitis C. Combination of alpha-lipoic acid (thioctic acid), silymarin and selenium. Three Case Histories. *Medizinische Klinik.* 94: 84-89, 1999.

Blumenthal M, Goldberg A, Brinckmann J., ed. Artichoke leaf. In *Herbal Medicine. Expanded Commission E Monographs.* Austin, Tex: American Botanical Council; Integrative Medicine Communications. 10-12, 2000.

Blumenthal M, Goldberg A, Brinckmann J., ed. Milk thistle fruit. In *Herbal Medicine. Expanded Commission E Monographs*. Austin, Texas: American Botanical Council; Integrative Medicine Communications. 257-263, 2000.

Blumenthal M, Goldberg A, Brinckmann J., ed Turmeric Root. In *Herbal Medicine: Expanded Commission E Monographs*. In *Herbal Medicine. Expanded Commission E Monographs*. Austin, Texas: American Botanical Council; Integrative Medicine Communications. 379-384, 2000.

Braaten JT, Wood PJ, Scott FW, et al. Oat beta-glucan reduces blood cholesterol concentration in hypercholesterolemic subjects. *European Journal of Clinical Nutrition*. 48:465-474, 1994.

Brown DJ. Milk thistle. *In Herbal Prescriptions for Health & Healing*. Twin Lakes, WI: Lotus Press. 193-202, 2000.

Camarasa J, Laguna JC, Gaspar A. Biochemical and histological pattern of cyanarin and caffeic acid treatment in CCL4 induced hepatoxicity. *Medical Science Research*. 15:91-92, 1987.

Carducci R, Armellina MF, Volpe C, et al. Silibinin and acute poisoning with Amanita phalloides. *Minerva Anestesiologica*. 62:187-193, 1996.

Cronin JR. Sulforaphane: Broccoli's chemoprotective secret. *Alternative and Complementary Therapies*. 6:149-151, 2000.

Dalvi RR. Alterations in hepatic phase I and Phase II biotransformation enzymes by garlic oil in rates. *Toxicology Letters*. 13: 1921-1923, 1992.

Daly AK, Cholerton S, Gregory W, et al. Metabolic polymorphisms. *Pharmacology & Therapeutics*. 57:129-160, 1993.

Dawson AH, Henry DA, McEwen J. Adverse reactions to N-acetylcysteine during treatment for paracetamol poisoning. *Medical Journal of Australia*. 150:329–331, 1989.

De Flora S, Bennicelli C, Camoirano A, et al. In vivo effects of N-acetylcysteine on glutathione metabolism and the biotransformation of carcinogenic and/or mutagenic compounds. *Carcinogenesis*. 6:1735-1745, 1985.

De Vries N, De Flora S. N-acetyl-l-cysteine. *Journal of Cellular Biochemistry*. 17F:S270-S277, 1993.

Dvorak Z, Kosina P, Walterova D, et al. Primary cultures of human hepatocytes as a tool in cytotoxicity studies: cell protection against model toxins by flavonolignans obtained from *Silybum marianum*. *Toxicology Letters*. 137:210-212, 2003.

Dwivedi C, Heck WJ, Downie AA, et al. Effect of calcium glucarate on beta-glucuronidase activity and glucarate content of certain vegetables and fruits. *Biochemical Medicine and Metabolic Biology.* 43:83-92, 1990.

Ernster L, Dallner G. Biochemical, physiological and medical aspects of ubiquinone function. *Biochimica et Biophysica Acta.* 1271:195-204, 1995.

Fleming T, ed. Artichoke. *In PDR® for Herbal Medicines.* Montvale, NJ: Medical Economics Company. 44-46, 2000.

Fleming T, ed. Dandelion. In *PDR® for Herbal Medicines.* Montvale, NJ: Medical Economics Company. 245-246, 2000.

Fleming T, ed. Licorice. *In PDR® for Herbal Medicines.* Montvale, NJ: Medical Economics Company. 469-474, 2000.

Fleming T, ed. Milk thistle. In *PDR® for Herbal Medicines.* Montvale, NJ: Medical Economics Company. 516-520, 2000.

Gebhardt R. Prevention of taurolithocholate-induced hepatic bile canalicular distortions by HPLC-characterized extracts of artichoke (Cynara scolymus) leaves. *Planta Medica.* 68:776-779, 2002.

Ghotra B, Vasanthan T, Temeli F. Tarurocholate absorption efficacy of Viscofiber and its blends with other commercial soluble fibers. Unpublished study, University of Edmonton, Cevena Bioproducts, 2004.

Hutt AJ, Caldwell J. Amino acid conjugation. In. *Conjugation Reactions In Drug Metabolism.* New York: Taylor & Francis. 273-305, 1990.

Kanter MZ. Comparison of oral and IV. N- acetylcysteine in the treatment of acetaminophen poisoning. *American Journal of Health System Pharmacy.* 63:1821, 2006.

Kerckhoffs DA, Brouns F, Hornstra G, et al. Effects on the human serum lipoprotein profile of betaglucan, soy protein and isoflavones, plant sterols and stanols, garlic and tocotrienols. *Journal of Nutrition.* 132:2494-2505, 2002.

Klaassen CD. Amdur MO, Doull J. *Casarett and Doull's Toxicology: The Basic Science of Poisons.* New York,: McGraw-Hill Health Professions Division. 163-168, 1996.

Kudryavtseva MV, Stein GI, Shashkov BV, Kudryavtsev BN. Functional activity of human hepatocytes under traumatic disease. *Experimental and Toxicological Pathology.* 50:53-57, 1998.

Lia A, Hallmans G, Sandberg AS, et al. Oat beta-glucan increases bile acid excretion and a fiber-rich barley fraction increases cholesterol excretion in ileostomy subjects. *American Journal of Clinical Nutrition.* 62:1245-1251, 1995.

Lynch RM, Robertson R., Anaphylactoid reactions to intravenous N-acetylcysteine: a prospective case controlled study. *Accident and Emergency Nursing.* 12:10–15, 2004.

Marlett JA, Hosig KB, Vollendorf NW, et al. Mechanism of serum cholesterol reduction by oat bran. *Hepatology.* 20:1450-1457, 1994.

Mislow K, Meluch WC. The stereochemistry of α-Lipoic acid. *Journal of the American Chemical Society.* 78: 2341–2342, 1956.

Nestle M. Broccoli sprouts in cancer prevention. *Nutrition Review.* 56:127-130, 1998.

Parodi O, De Chiara B, Baldassarre D, et al. Plasma cysteine and glutathione are independent markers of postmethionine load endothelial dysfunction. *Clinical Biochemistry.* 40: 188-193, 2007.

Person JR, Bernhard JD. Autointoxication revisited. *Journal of the American Academy of Dermatology.* 15:559-563, 1986.

Piper JT, Singhal SS, Salameh MS, et al. Mechanisms of anticarcinogenic properties of curcumin: the effect of curcumin on glutathione linked detoxification enzymes in rat liver. *International Journal of Biochemistry and Cell Biology.* 30:445-456, 1998.

Porth CM. The liver and hepatobiliary system. In *Pathophysiology: Concepts of Altered Health States.* 5th ed. Philadelphia, PA: Lippincott. 745-753, 1998.

Reed LJ, DeBusk BG, Gunsalus IC, et al. Crystalline alpha-lipoic acid; a catalytic agent associated with pyruvate dehydrogenase. *Science.* 114: 93–94, 1951.

Ringman JM, Frautshy SA, Cole GM, et al. A potential role of the curry spice curcumin in Alzheimer's disease. *Current Alzheimer's Research.* 2:131-136, 2005.

Saenz Rodriguez T, Garcia Gimenez D, et al. Choleretic activity and biliary elimination of lipids and bile acids induced by an artichoke leaf extract in rats. *Phytomedicine.* 9:687-693, 2002.

Saller R, Meier R, Brignoli R. The use of silymarin in the treatment of liver diseases. *Drugs.* 61:2035-2063, 2001.

Smith RL, Williams RT. History of the discovery of the conjugation mechanisms. In *Metabolic Conjugation And Metabolic Hydrolysis.* New York: Academic Press, Inc. 1-19, 1970.

Susan M. Rao MN. Induction of glutathione S-transferase activity by curcumin in mice. *Arzneimittelforschung.* 42:962-964, 1992.

Valenzuela A, Aspillaga M, Vial S, et al. Selectivity of silymarin on the increase of the glutathione content in different tissues of the rat. *Planta Medica.* 55:420-422, 1989.

Vogel G, Tuchweber B, Trost W, et al. Protection by silibinin against Amanita phalloides intoxication in beagles. *Toxicology and Applied Pharmacology.* 73:355-362, 1984.

Williams AC, Cartright LS, Ramsden DB. Parkinson's disease: the first common neurological disease due to auto-intoxication? *QJM.* 98:215-226, 2005.

Chapter 8

Aasath J, Jacobsen J, Andersen O, et al. Treatment of mercury and lead poisonings with dimercaptosuccinic acid (DMSA) and sodium dimercaptopropanesulfonate (DMPS). *Analyst.* 120: 853ff , 1995.

Aposhian HV, Aposhian MM. Meso-2,3-dimercaptosuccinic acid: Chemical, pharmacological and toxicological properties of an orally effective metal chelating agent. *Annual Review of Pharmacology and Toxicology.* 30: 279–306, 1990.

Flickstein A. Healthmate infrared saunas, *Townsend Letter for Doctors*, 202:66-70, 2000.

Gard.R, Brown EJ. History of sauna/hyperthermia; Past and present efficacy in detoxification. *Townsend Letter for Doctors.* June 1992:470-478, July 1992:650-660, Oct. 1992:846-854, Aug-Sept 1999:76-86.

Inoue S, Kabaya m. 1989, Biological activities caused by far infrared radiation, *International Journal of Biometeorology.* 33:145-150, 1989.

Johnson-Restrepo B, Kannan K, Rapaport D P, et al.. Polybrominated diphenyl ethers and polychlorinated biphenyls in human adipose tissue from New York. *Environmental Science & Technology.* 39: 5177–5182, 2005.

Krop J, Chemical sensitivity after intoxication at work with solvents: response to sauna therapy. *Journal of Alternative and Complementary Medicine.* 4:77-86, 1998.

Naert C, Piette M, Bruneel N, et al. Occurrence of polychlorinated biphenyls and polybrominated diphenyl ethers in Belgian human adipose tissue samples. *Archives of Environmental Contamination and Toxicology.* 50: 290–296, 2006.

Pizzorno, JE, Murray, MT. *Textbook of Natural Medicine*, 3rd edition, London: Churchill Livingstone, 2005.

Rea WJ, Pan Y, Johnson AR. Clearing of toxic volatile hydrocarbons from humans. *Boletín de la Asociación Médica de Puerto Rico.* 83:321-324, 1991.

Rogers SA, *Tired or Toxic.* Syracuse, NY: Prestige Publishers, 1990.

Rooney J. The role of thiols, dithiols, nutritional factors and interacting ligands in the toxicology of mercury. *Toxicology.* 234:145–156, 2007.

Schnare DW, Ben M, Shields MG. Body burden reductions of PCBs, PBBs and chlorinated pesticides in human subjects. *Ambio.* 13:378-380, 1984.

The Toxome Project. Health effects of pollutants found in people. Available at www.ewg.org/sites/ humantoxome.

Chapter 9

Abrams S, Griffin I, Hawthorne K, et al. A combination of prebiotic short- and long-chain inulin-type fructans enhances calcium absorption and bone mineralization in young adolescents. *American Journal of Clinical Nutrition.* 82: 471-476, 2005.

Anderson JW, <u>Allgood LD</u>, <u>Lawrence A</u>, et al. Cholesterol-lowering effects of psyllium intake adjunctive to diet therapy in men and women with hypercholesterolemia: Meta-analysis of 8 controlled trials. *American Journal of Clinical Nutrition,* 71: 472–479, 2000.

Block, E. The chemistry of garlic and onions. *Scientific American.*252: 114–119, 1995.

Block, E. The organosulfur chemistry of the genus Allium — implications for organic sulfur chemistry. *Angewandte Chemie International Edition.* 104: 1158–1203, 1992.

Brooks JD, Paton VG, Vidanes G. Potent induction of phase 2 enzymes in human prostate cells by sulforaphane. *Cancer Epidemiology, Biomarkers and Prevention.* 10: 949–954, 2001.

Coudray C, Demigné C, Rayssiguier Y. Effects of dietary fibers on magnesium absorption in animals and humans. *Journal of Nutrition.* 133: 1-4, 2003.

Eastwood MA, Brydon WG, Tadesse K. Effect of fiber on colon function. In *Medical Aspects of Dietary Fiber.* New York: Plenum Press. 1-26, 1980.

Fiber Health Claims That Meet Significant Scientific Agreement, US Food and Drug Administration. Available at www.cfsan.fda.gov/~dms/lab-ssa.html.

Fuchs, CS, Giovannucci EL, Colditz GA, et al. Dietary fiber and the risk of colorectal cancer and adenoma in women. *New England Journal of Medicine.* 340:169-176, 1999.

Grodner M, Anderson SL, DeYoung S. Fiber. In *Foundations and Clinical Applications of Nutrition: A Nursing Approach.* St. Louis, MO: Mosby. 102-108, 2000.

Hallfrisch J, Scholfield D, Behall K. Glucose and insulin responses to a new zero-energy fiber source. *Journal of the American College of Nutrition.* 21:410-415, 2002.

Higgins JA. Resistant starch: metabolic effects and potential health benefits. *Journal of AOAC International.* 87:761-767, 2004.

Lau BH. Detoxifying radioprotective and phagocyte-enhancing effects of garlic. *International Clinical Nutrition Review.* 9, 1:27-31, 1989.

Le HT , Schaldach CM, Firestone GL, et al. Plant-derived 3,3'-Diindolylmethane is a strong androgen antagonist in human prostate cancer cells. *The Journal of Biological Chemistry.* 278:21136-21145, 2003.

Li G, et al. Antiproliferative effects of garlic constituents on cultured human breast cancer cells. *Oncology Report.* 2:787-791, 1995.

Marlett JA, Kajs TM, Fischer MH. An unfermented gel component of psyllium seed husk promotes laxation as a lubricant in humans. *American Journal of Clinical Nutrition.* 72:784-789, 2000.

Prynne CJ, Southgate DAT. The effects of a supplement of dietary fibre on faecal excretion by human subjects. *British Journal of Nutrition.* 41:495-503, 1979.

Sumiyoshi H, Wargovich MJ. Chemoprevention of 1,2-dimethylhydrazine-induced colon cancer in mice by naturally occurring organosulfur compounds. *Cancer Research.* 50:5084-5087, 1990.

Tadi PP, Teel RW, Lau BHS. Organosulfur compounds of garlic modulate mutagenesis, metabolism, and DNA binding of aflatoxin B1. *Nutrition and Cancer.* 15:87-95, 1991.

Tungland BC, Meyer D. Nondigestible oligo- and polysaccharides (dietary fiber): their physiology and role in human health and food. *Comprehensive Reviews in Food Science and Food Safety* 1:73-92, 2002.

Wargovich MJ. Diallyl sulfide, a flavor component of garlic (Allium sativum), inhibits dimethylhydrazine-induced colon cancer. *Carcinogenesis.* 8:487-489, 1987.

Chapter 10

Beck S, Olek A, Walter J. From genomics to epigenomics: a loftier view of life. *Nature Biotechnology.* 17:1144, 1999.

Fraga MF, Ballestar E, Paz MF, et al. Epigenetic differences arise during the lifetime of monozygotic twins. *Proceedings of the National Academy of Sciences USA.* 102: 10604–10609, 2005.

Hall J G, Lopez-Rangel, E. *Twins and Twinning,* New York: Churchill Livingstone. *395*-404, 1966.

Jones PA, Martienssen R. A blueprint for a Human Epigenome Project: the AACR Human Epigenome Workshop. *Cancer Research.* 65, 11241–11246, 2005.

Sharpe RM, Irvine DS. How strong is the evidence of a link between environmental chemicals and adverse effects on human reproductive health? *British Medical Journal.* 328:447-451, 2004.

Watters E. DNA Is Not Destiny. *Discover Magazine.* 75:32-37, November 2006.

Chapter 11

Baille-Hamilton PF. Chemical toxins: a hypothesis to explain the global obesity epidemic. *Journal of Alternative and Complementary Medicine.* 8:185–192, 2002.

Baptista T. Body weight gain induced by antipsychotic drugs: Mechanisms and management. *Acta psychiatrica Scandinavica.*100:3–16, 1999.

Dar E, Kanarek MS, Anderson HA, et al. Fish consumption and reproductive outcomes in Green Bay, Wisconsin. *Environmental Research.* 59:189–201, 1992.

Deichmann WB, MacDonald WE, Cubit DA, et al. Effects of starvation in rats with elevated DDT and dieldrin tissue levels. *Internationales Archiv für Arbeitsmedizin.* 29: 233–252, 1972.

Flegal KM, Carroll MD, Kuczmarski RJ, et al. Overweight and obesity in the United States: Prevalence and trends, 1960–1994. *International Journal of Obesity and Related Metabolic Disorders.* 22:39-47, 1998.

Heindel JJ. Endocrine disruptors and the obesity epidemic. *Toxicology Sciences.* 76:247-249, 2003.

Mead MN. Origins of obesity. *Environmental Health Perspectives.* 112:A344, 2004.

Seegal RF, Bush B, Brosch KO. Decreases in dopamine concentrations in adult, non-human primate brain persist following removal from polychlorinated biphenyls. *Toxicology.* 86:71–87, 1994.

Takahama K, Ishii J, Kanda M. Toxicological studies on organochlorine pesticides: Effect of long term administration of organochlorine pesticides on rabbit weight and organ weight. *Nippon Hoigaku Zasshi.* 26:5–10, 1972.

Wang G-J, Volkow ND, Logan J, et al. Brain dopamine and obesity. *Lancet.* 357:354–357, 2001.

Chapter 12

Rogers SA. Chemical sensitivity: Breaking the paralyzing paradigm. *Internal Medicine World Report.* March 15-31: 8-31, 1992.

Roundtree R. The use of phytochemicals in the biotransformation and elimination of environmental toxins. *Medicines from the Earth 2003: Official Proceedings.* Gaia Herbal Research Institute, Brevard, N.C. 115-128, 2003.

INDEX

A

Acetylation, 98
Air
    filters, 126
    toxins in, 48–50
Alpha lipoic acid, 134
Aluminum, 76
Alzheimer's disease, 13
Amino acid conjugation, 98
Antacids, 106, 120
Antioxidants, 77–78, 129, 165–66
Arsenic, 22, 53–54
Artichokes, 132–33, 167
ATP (adenosine triphosphate), 31, 59, 130
Atrazine, 8, 73
Attention deficit disorder (ADD), 5
Autism, 5, 69
Autoimmune diseases, 113, 114

B

Beets, 167
Beta-glucans, 160
Bile, 93, 99–100, 107, 117, 129, 167, 187
Blood-letting, 27
BMI (body mass index), 179–82
Body
    accumulation of chemicals in, 15, 25, 30-31, 39–41
    number of cells in, 15, 31
    self-healing abilities of, 10–12, 18–19

Body burden
    definition of, 16, 23, 58, 151
    determining, 23
    equation for, 24, 151
    estimates of, 16, 24, 137–38
    factors influencing, 23
    reducing, 58–59, 68, 152, 191
Bottled water, 35–37
BPA (bisphenol A), 15, 17, 40, 43–44, 83
Breath, 91–92

C

Cadmium, 63–64, 135
Calcium, 60, 71–72
Cancer
    environment and, 12–13, 15, 16, 69, 74–75, 88
    prevalence of, 5
Carbamates, 67
Cardiovascular disease, 5, 12–13
Carpeting, 49, 199
Carson, Rachel, 7, 38, 66, 73, 83
CCA (chromated copper arsenate), 54
CDG (calcium D-glucarate), 134
Cells
    composition of, 31, 32
    definition of, 31
    energy production by, 31–32
    number of, in the body, 15, 31
Cellular respiration, 32
Chelation, 146–50
Chemical load. See Body burden
Chemicals. See also Pollution; Toxins

accumulation of, in the body, 15, 26, 30–31, 39–41
environmentally persistent, 42
impact of, 17, 20–22, 26
new, 16
registered by the EPA, 15–16
testing of, 15–16, 17, 43, 55
ubiquity of, 15, 37–38, 44–45
Children
cancer in, 69
endocrine disruptors and, 84
lead and, 60–61
obesity in, 177
playground equipment for, 53–54
Cholesterol, 162
Chromosomes, 13, 14, 170, 172
Citrus fruits, 167
Cleaning products, 67–68, 125, 199–200
Colon, 108
Colonics, 33
Compliance, importance of, 20
Constipation, 108
CoQ10, 130, 134
Cytochrome P450 system, 96–97

D

Dandelion root, 133, 167
DDT, 7–8, 24, 40, 57, 66, 83
Dental fillings, 63
DES (diethylstilbestrol), 83–84
Detoxification. See also Whole body cleansing
criteria for, 28
critics of, 28–29
definitions of, 25–26
excretory pathways for, 91–101
history of, 27–28
improper approaches to, 27, 33–34, 124
learning about, 18, 19
myths about, 27, 29–30
overview of, 30–34
Phase I, 95–97, 129, 134
Phase II, 92, 95–96, 97–99, 134
physical appearance and, 26, 32
science of, 33–34, 123–36
tools for, 19
DGL (deglycyrrhizinated licorice), 119–20, 128

Diabetes, 5, 13, 65, 69, 80, 198
Diet
fad, 184–85
historic changes in, 109–10
keys to healthy, 194
Western, 109, 110
Digestion. See also GI (gastrointestinal) tract
problems with, 112–15
process of, 105–8
Digestive enzymes, 118–19, 127
DIM (diindolylmethane), 99, 204
Dioxins, 83, 141
DMSA (2,3-dimercaptosuccinic acid), 142, 147–50
DNA
environment and, 12–15, 72
function of, 13–14
Human Genome Project, 169–73
structure of, 170–71
Drugs, 138
Duodenum, 105, 106, 107

E

Eczema, 13
EDTA (ethylenediamine tetra-acetic acid), 146–47
Education, importance of, 19
Ellagic acid, 167
Endocrine disruptors, 81–85, 88
Enemas, 27–28, 33
Energy production, 31–32, 130
Enteric nervous system, 104
Environment. See also Pollution
biological, 71–72
genetics and, 12–15, 72, 175–76
role of, in health, 18–19, 70–72, 74–75
Environmental Protection Agency (EPA), 15, 54, 56, 67–68, 140
Environmental Working Group (EWG), 36–37, 39–40, 53–54, 55
Enzymes, 59, 96, 118–19, 127
Epigenetics, 13, 173–76
Esophagus, 105
Estrogen
chemicals mimicking, 17, 44, 84, 88
metabolites, 99
Ethylphenol, 141
Exercise, 101, 142–45

ABOUT THE AUTHOR

Gaetano A. Morello, ND, received his doctorate in naturopathic medicine from Bastyr University. His bachelor of science degree in cell biology and nutrition is from the University of British Columbia in Vancouver, BC. Dr. Morello is a board member of the Association of Naturopathic Physicians of British Columbia, the British Columbia Association of Naturopathic Physicians, and the Canadian Association of Naturopathic Physicians. He is a member of the New York Academy of Sciences and a member of the scientific advisory board of Schwabe North America and Enzymatic Therapy International, a major manufacturer of nutritional and herbal supplements. He is a contributing author to A Textbook of Natural Medicine, the most definitive text on natural medicine in the world. Over the past 17 years, Dr. Morello has written hundreds of articles, given more than 1,000 medical presentations throughout the world, and has done numerous radio and television interviews throughout North America. Dr. Morello is regarded as a leading authority on the topic of natural medicine. For more information and useful resources, visit www.drgaetano.com.